At the
BREAKING POINT
of HISTORY

How Decades of U.S. Duplicity
Enabled the Pandemic

JANET PHELAN

Back-cover author photo: ©Carlos Johnson
Cover Art: ©Santiago P. Seoane

Published by:
Trine Day LLC
PO Box 577
Walterville, OR 97489
1-800-556-2012
www.TrineDay.com
trineday@icloud.com

Library of Congress Control Number: 2021941559

Phelan, Janet
At the Breaking Point of History—1st ed.
p. cm.
Epub (ISBN-13) 978-1-63424-369-8
Print (ISBN-13) 978-1-63424-368-1
1. National security -- United States. 2. COVID-19 (Disease) -- Political aspects
-- United States. 3. Epidemics -- Prevention. 4. COVID-19 (Disease) -- Social
aspects -- United States. 5. MEDICAL/Infectious Diseases. 6. POLITICAL
SCIENCE/American Government/National. I. Title

First Edition
10 9 8 7 6 5 4 3

Printed in the USA
Distribution to the Trade by:
Independent Publishers Group (IPG)
814 North Franklin Street
Chicago, Illinois 60610
312.337.0747
www.ipgbook.com

To Szmul Zygielbojm

Acclaim for Janet Phelan's books

Janet Phelan is a phenomenal, thrilling writer.
– Activist Post

Delivering on the widely acknowledged promise of her writing, Phelan produces another spellbinding work of investigative journalism
– Katherine Hine, *Columbus Free Press*, book review of Exile.

Stellar writer, factual investigative journalism, and heroine for exposing these concerns to humanity.
– Dr. Robert Duncan, DARPA / CIA scientist

Janet Phelan has been asking the right questions for a long time. It's time we start paying attention.
– Sean Stone, filmmaker and talk show host

I am so excited about this book Janet decided to write. It will be a god-send for many in these uncertain times. I am a fan of her work, I know her dogged dedication to accuracy and truth. She writes from her heart not only for the enlightenment of those seeking important information and wisdom therefrom, but she also writes for the overall betterment of the human condition.
– Karen Melton Stewart, NSA whistleblower

If there is one message that I want to leave with you today, based on my experience … is that there is no question that there will be a challenge to the coming administration in the arena of infectious diseases … there will be a surprise outbreak

– Dr. Anthony Fauci, January 2017

CONTENTS

PREFACE

Shortly after the events of September 2001, it became clear to me that a pandemic would be launched. There were a number of reasons for this perception. First, there were legal changes which gave the US government immunity for launching a pandemic. There were also changes in domestic law which served to completely occlude the hand of the government in creating or deploying this, criminalizing the release of information. The US, which is a party to the international treaty known as the Biological Weapons Convention, also began to heavily and consistently misrepresent her activities to the Convention at large.

Subsequent to the attacks of September 11, the anthrax attacks, dubbed AMERITHRAX, were launched. The letters laced with anthrax, sent to media and to members of Congress, served to expand the US's biological weapons programs through increased funding, the amount and purposes of which have also been occluded from public oversight and awareness.

By chance, I stumbled upon an engineering project which would serve as a covert delivery system for a bio or chem attack. As I began to document this, largely focusing on blueprints of the system in question, I was forced to flee the US.

For the past fifteen years, my journalism has focused on the pending pandemic – Who, What, Where, When and How. These articles have appeared in Activist Post and, for several years, in New Eastern Outlook and elsewhere. Under the mantle of an NGO that I created in 2010, I also twice traveled to Geneva, Switzerland and brought these concerns to the attention of the Biological Weapons Convention.

Today, we find ourselves in the midst of a pandemic, one which has collapsed economies, caused death by starvation and has resulted in severe new restrictions on civil rights in the US and elsewhere. Numerous medical professionals and researchers are questioning the genesis of the Covid-19 agent, whether or not it was bioengineered and deliberately released and also questioning the course taken to shut down whole countries and demand that people stay at home. Questions have also been raised as to the verifiability of the numbers alleged to have died from this novel coronavirus, pointing to dictates from the CDC to list deaths not directly caused by the virus as virus-caused deaths.

In the middle of this chaos, these articles, many of which were written long before the pandemic, point to a plan to launch one. As the country begins to reopen, the trajectory of these articles should evoke grave concern for the future.

It is, however, not too late to act. Armed with the information compiled and reported on here, we still can move forward to save ourselves and save our world. But first, we need to understand the nature of the threat.

FOREWORD

This book is divided into five sections, each containing previously published articles arranged around a theme. Some of the articles have been edited for this project, others are in the same format in which they were first published. The first section, SOME BACKGROUND, provides some context for the reader as to activities involving the US which constitute gross and continued violations of bioweapons norms.

The first article in this section, The BWC Turns 40, provides a sense of the history of the US's bioweapons programs .The US has insisted on the misnomer of "biodefense" to describe her programs, and this article and subsequent articles in this section provide a more realistic history of the US's activities in this field.

These activities include the US being caught mailing live anthrax to over 194 labs worldwide. They include concerns raised by other countries that the US has an active bioweapons program. Intimations by those in the know that a pandemic is in the works are also discussed in the articles in this section, as are some of the more concerning actions taken by the multinational corporations, Bayer and Monsanto. As illustrative of the US's propensity to ignore the rights of test subjects, an article on the EPA and chemical weapons testing is also included.

The second section, THE STATE OF THE SCIENCE, focuses on genetics and genetic weapons. Genetics has become prominent in weapons development, due to the possibility of these weapons affecting only certain races or specified individuals. As it is a primary contention of this author that there is a genetic obsession that is unfolding in the policies of the US, the efforts to refine these agents are of particular interest. CREEPING TOWARDS FASCISM admittedly contains a hodge podge of articles, from those discussing current efforts involving non- consensual human experimentation and torture to evidence that a cure for cancer may already exist, to anthrax experiments conducted courtesy of US anthrax stockpiles. The wide sweep of this section is intended to provide more substantiation to the allegations that the US is in defiance of human rights norms as well as international accords involving weapons testing and stockpiling.

The fourth section, BIOWEAPONS: AT THE BREAKING POINT OF HISTORY, includes articles intended to show that the progression of these activities is clearly becoming a risk to the world. This section also contains articles, such as Dancing the Apocalypso with the Microbial Gestapo and US Lies to the UN, which highlight the legal violations committed by the US government in her pursuit of an opaque but increasingly all too apparent bioweapons agenda.

The fifth and final section, THE PANDEMIC, brings us up to the present. Special attention is given in this section to the revelations of the nature of water as a potential selective pandemic delivery system as well as how the Covid pandemic may eventuate into a staging platform for genocide.

The EPILOGUE attempts to put the pandemic crisis into a frame revealing global imperatives.

There is, naturally, another section, as yet unwritten. It could be titled AFTERWORD or even AFTERMATH. It is the author's hope, that by publishing this book, such a section may become unnecessary. Every recent generation has experienced a crisis in runaway governance, whether it be in Germany or in Russia, China or even in the US. By seeking to clarify the current situation, it may be possible to derail the otherwise inevitable. For, as the title article to this book declares, *"The signs pointing to future deployments are everywhere now. The only question remaining is will we awaken to history before history ends."*

I would like to thank those who have supported and encouraged this work. Specifically, I would like to thank Michael Edwards at Activist Post for publishing many of these initial articles. I would like to thank Kovil Helm, who edited a number of the articles and also provided helpful input as to the structuring of this book. Thanks also to the numerous individuals who contacted me with details of infrastructure work in their own cities and to the military officers, present and former, who provided me with details as to military activities which enhanced my knowledge of this issue. A special thanks to Eben Rey, formerly at KPFK, who gave me my very first opportunity to discuss these issues on air, and to Frank Allen, formerly with Republic Broadcasting Network, who has given me a virtual carte blanche to discuss on air these concerns and much more.

Through the years, the support and encouragement of a number of radio show hosts, too numerous to mention, have propelled this work forward. You know who you are and even though you remain unnamed here, my heartfelt thanks goes out to you all.

Finally, to Karen Melton Stewart and Ben Colodzin, for the hours spent on the phone with me, as I passed through discouragement into renewal, the deepest appreciation.

SOME BACKGROUND

1

THE BIOLOGICAL WEAPONS CONVENTION TURNS 40 – ARE WE ANY SAFER?

This year, the Biological Weapons Convention (BWC) celebrated its 40th birthday in Geneva, at the Palais Nacions. Amidst speeches and backslapping within the coterie of the BWC crowd, the question that hangs in the air is – Are we really any safer?

The Biological Weapons Convention was signed by the three depositary countries – Russia, Great Britain and the United States – in 1972 and entered into force in 1975. The announcement by the Nixon administration in 1969 that the US would unilaterally renounce the use of biological weapons and discontinue its biological weapons program provided an impetus towards the establishment of the treaty.

IS THIS A TREATY OR WHAT?

Unlike other disarmament treaties, the BWC has no verification protocol. What this means is that there is no way for the Convention to check to see if those who have signed and ratified the Convention are in fact abiding by its dictates.

In 2001, after several years of meetings and consultations, an Ad Hoc Committee presented to the Convention a verification protocol for approval. Led by John Bolton, the US delegation walked out, boycotting the protocol. Due to the refusal of the US to approve the verification mechanisms, the BWC remains a paper tiger. It is, in reality, a treaty in name only, with no way to check on compliance and no way to deal with violations.

The US team boycotted the protocol only months before the attacks of September 11 and the subsequent anthrax attacks. Based on what turned out to be false statements that Iraq was hosting an offensive biological weapons program, the US invaded Iraq in 2003. The FBI subsequently allocated responsibility for the anthrax attacks to a Fort Detrick researcher, Dr. Bruce Ivins, who conveniently committed suicide on the eve of his probable arrest. Subsequent reports have cast doubt on the likelihood that Ivins was the culprit.[1] In fact, the weaponized anthrax very likely came from a Battelle lab or from Dugway Proving Ground in Utah.

Battelle is a private non-profit which also manages US Department of Energy and Homeland Security labs. Dugway Proving Ground is a military base. Both a Battelle lab in Ohio and Dugway had anthrax from the very same vial that Dr. Ivins had access to at Ft. Detrick and which was determined to contain the weaponized anthrax used in the anthrax attacks. In other words, the anthrax most likely came from a facility funded by the US government.

The FBI declined to investigate personnel at either of these other facilities.

Later assertions, which turned out also to be highly questionable, concerning chemical weapons deployment by Syria in August of 2013, prompted the Obama administration to call for war against Syria that year. This was derailed by the diplomatic efforts of Mr. Putin, who arranged for Syria to become a party to the Chemical Weapons Convention. At that point, further accusations began to mount concerning a purported Syrian bioweapons program.

Parenthetically, the US had also falsely accused the former Soviet Union of using biological weapons in Afghanistan, Laos and Cambodia. The "yellow rain" controversy, as it came to be known, was eventually resolved and the Soviet Union exonerated of the accusations.

According to *The Future of Biological Weapons Revisited*, by Koos van der Bruggen and Barend ter Haar, the lack of a verification protocol is only one issue plaguing the BWC. Other concerns about enforcing compliance remain.

The authors also cite concerns that the science going into the production of these sorts of weapons has advanced far beyond the reach of the BWC. In addition, there is a continued and uneasy debate concerning the "dual use" issue. Put plainly, it is necessary to have the biological agent – weapon–at hand in order to produce a countermeasure. This purportedly defensive aspect of bioweapons research opens the door, and opens it widely, to offensive capabilities.

Hey Buddy, What'd you do with that vial?

Our collective safety depends on a number of factors. The proliferation of labs – there are now over 1350 such level 3 research labs in the US alone– has resulted in an increasing incidence of accidents. As reported in a 2014 USA Today article, US labs mishandled dangerous biomaterials at least 1100 times between 2008-2012.[2]

These are only the reported numbers. As discussed in Kenneth King's 2010 book, *Germs Gone Wild*, there have surfaced numerous incidents wherein a lab accident, involving release or illness, was hastily covered up.

Richard Ebright, a biosafety expert at Rutgers University, has stated that there are more than four events each week which could be described as a loss or release of bioweapons materials from US labs.

Accidents are one concern. Another concern would be intentional release.

The US's Illegal Bioweapons Program

The manipulation of false BW assertions by the United States does not end with attempts to invade other countries. Valid questions have arisen as to whether the US is, in fact, engaged in a secret BW program of its own.

Information buttressing concerns that the US has, in fact, launched a secret biological weapons program was turned over to the Biological Weapons Convention at the Seventh Review Conference in 2011. This reporter traveled to Geneva in December of 2011 and put this statement on the record.[3]

The information provided the delegates, both in a short speech and in subsequent handouts, reflected the following concerns:

- The United States has amended its biological weapons legislation via Section 817 of the US PATRIOT Act and is now giving its own agents immunity from prosecution for violating the law.

- The United States has failed to report this change in legislation to the BWC, as it is mandated to do in a politically binding agreement.

- These weapons are reported to be secretly stockpiled at Sierra Army Depot in Northern California

- Two separate domestic delivery systems have been delineated – one involving country-wide reconfigurations of water systems, and the other involving impostor pharmaceuticals. Both delivery systems are capable of selective, demographic targeting – either of pre-selected individuals or, by extension, those who comprise a particular group.

The text of Section 817, with the problematic portion highlighted, follows: Whoever knowingly violates this section shall be fined as provided in this title, imprisoned not more than 10 years, or both, but *the prohibition contained in this section shall not apply with respect to any duly authorized United States governmental activity.*

Following the presentation to the Convention at large, this reporter then contacted officials with Disarmament Affairs at the United Nations, in an effort to turn over further supporting documentation substantiating the allegations that the US has developed a covert delivery system, country wide, for a water-borne BW attack. The documentation contained blueprints of water systems, correspondence with multiple government agencies and more.

The response by the officials with Disarmament Affairs was similar to that of someone being subjected to a strong electric current: Shock and aversion.

As reported in this reporter's summary article from the Convention:[4]

> Valere Mantels, political officer for the Geneva branch of the UN disarmament affairs, refused to accept further documentation, stating "I am not going to burn my hands by turning over documentation to the Secretary General." Peter Kolarov of Disarmament Affairs declined to meet with this reporter, suggesting the documentation be taken to New York (?). UN Political officer, Bantan Nugroho, also of Disarmament Affairs, did agree to a meeting and was handed a stack of relevant documentation. He declined to take action…
>
> A final meeting with Jarmo Sareva, Director of Disarmament Affairs at the Geneva branch of the United Nations, ended in a stalemate when he informed this reporter, "We are neutral. We do not take sides." When it was suggested that neutrality was a concept useful when there was a debate about facts, but here the documentation amassed may have transcended what could be termed a "difference of opinion," he mumbled something about how countries might "use this information for political purposes…." This reporter pushed ahead, stating that "we are not talking about missing money here. We are talking about the possible destruction of human life on a nearly unimaginable scale."
>
> When Sareva did not respond this reporter terminated the meeting.

In the intervening years since the Seventh Review Conference of the BWC, concerns have increased in many sectors that that the US has launched a secret biological weapons program with intent to deploy.

One continuing concern revolves around the evasive behavior by the US in terms of reporting its bioweapons activities. The US is mandated by a politically binding agreement to report changes in its bioweapons legislation to the Convention at large. According to Chris Park, Director of Biological Policy with the State Department and a delegate to the BWC, the US "forgot" to report the changes in the problematic Section 817.

That was a fairly big "Oops." The changes to the US's biological weapons laws essentially removed the US from compliance with the BWC. The US would therefore have every reason in the world to attempt to obscure this from the Convention members.

Concerns that bioweapons may be deployed to specifically devastate pre-selected demographic groups were enhanced in the recent Ebola crisis. Ebola broke out in the areas in which BSLs (biosafety labs) already were in place. There are such labs located in Monrovia, Liberia; Kenema, Sierra Leone; and two in Guinea. These countries were all hit hard with Ebola. Either concurrent accidents or intentional releases could have resulted in the subsequent devastation visited upon these countries by the Ebola virus.

Wink Wink, Nod Nod

Numerous insiders, with the military, government and vaccine companies, have publicly stated the imminent nature of either a bioweapons attack or a pandemic (how would we know the difference unless we were told?). Those making these predictions include former US Senators Talent and Graham, now of the WMD center in Washington, DC; Dr. Daniel Gerstein Department of Homeland Security's Deputy Under Secretary for Science & Technology; Dr. Robert Kadlec, whose resume includes such high-level positions as Special Assistant To the President and Senior Director/Biodefense Policy, Special Assistant To the President/Homeland Security and Colonel in the USAF; and vaccine manufacturer J. Joseph Kim, to name a few.

Most recently, the British newspaper The Guardian joined the choir, abandoning reportage and instead evidencing a gift for prophecy in the following headline: "Ebola isn't the big one. So what is? And are we ready for it?"

At the time this story ran, October 3, 2014, no one else was quite sure that Ebola wasn't "the big one." One would wonder when The Guardian began prognosticating…

In an interview in *GQ* in 2007, former Secretary of State Colin Powell made the following assertion:

> "What is the greatest threat facing us now? People will say it's terrorism. But are there any terrorists in the world who can change the American way of life or our political system? No. Can they knock down a building? Yes. Can they kill somebody? Yes. But can they change us? No. Only we can change ourselves…..The only thing that can really destroy us is us."[5]

> – May 25, 2015

2

THE ANTHRAX FILES: US FORCES CONDUCTED MULTIPLE SECRET ANTHRAX EXPERIMENTS IN SOUTH KOREA

The initial admission by the Department of Defense that one sample of live anthrax was inadvertently sent to Osan Air Base in South Korea has now been revealed to be grossly inaccurate.

According to a recent report by a US/South Korea joint working group, a US military defense laboratory at Dugway Proving Grounds mailed anthrax to South Korea at least *fifteen times* prior to the previously acknowledged March, 2015 delivery. These other anthrax samples were delivered to Yongsan Garrison, in central South Korea, between 2009 and 2014. In addition, a 1-milliliter sample of the *Yersinia pestis* bacterium (which can cause the bubonic plague) was sent along with the anthrax to Osan.

The United States has denied accusations that it lied in a May press release, which stated that:

> "The laboratory biological defense training, part of the Joint United States Forces Korea Portal and Integrated Threat Recognition Program at Osan Air Base, has been halted pending further review… This was the first time the training has been conducted."[6]

In an email reply to the Washington correspondent with Korean publication *JoongAng Daily*, Pentagon spokesman Bill Urban wrote:

> "Following the inadvertent delivery of potentially live *Bacillus anthracis*, the 51st Fighter Wing at Osan Air Base correctly informed the public in the Osan area that the shipment supported the first Joint U.S. Forces Korea Portal and Integrated Threat Recognition program's training at that location."

JoongAng went on to report that Urban suggested that the press release had been misunderstood and the intended meaning was that "the first time" training only referred to the first in Osan, not in all of South Korea.[7]

It has recently come to light that the Pentagon FedExed live anthrax to all fifty states and to nine foreign countries. The Department of Defense has declared that errors in the process of inactivating the anthrax resulted in the inadvertence wherein live anthrax was FedExed to foreign and domestic laboratories.

The joint working group has refused to discuss the amount of the anthrax samples used in Yongsan, citing "military secrets." The working group's conclusions are already under fire, with allegations being mounted that it relied too heavily on input from Washington.

Under current regulations, the US does not need to inform the South Korean government if it sends "inactive" germs. Since the recent crisis involving live anthrax being sent to South Korea and elsewhere, recommendations are being considered to change this practice to include advisories to foreign countries that biological materials are being shipped in, and for what purpose.

The US states that the anthrax sent to Osan was to be used to test protective gear. The US has consistently stated that North Korea maintains an offensive biological weapons program and is manufacturing weaponized anthrax and smallpox, among other agents, at a facility near Pyongyang

In response, the North Korean government has offered to throw open the doors of the Pyongyang plant and has invited the Americans in to check the facility, which North Korea states is a pesticide manufacturing plant. As reported in *The Guardian*, a spokesman for the North Korean National Defence Commission said,

> "Come here right now, with all the 535 members of the House of Representatives and the Senate as well as the imbecile secretaries and deputy secretaries of the government who have made their voices hoarse screaming for new sanctions."[8]

A report from US Undersecretary of Defense Frank Kendall concerning the DoD review of the laboratory procedures which resulted in the purported failure to inactivate the anthrax has raised further questions. Kendall states that Dugway Proving Grounds has had

> "a relatively high incidence (20%) of post-inactivation viability tests that showed unsuccessful inactivation, *but failed to address all the root causes of this high incidence.*" (emphasis added)

Kendall also makes a curious reference to an apparent intent behind the failure to inactivate anthrax at Dugway. He writes:

"I agree with the Review Committee that the combination of unique characteristics at DPG, to include high volume production, low sampling size, *intentionally impure products,* and more immediate post-inactivation viability testing are possible contributing factors."(emphasis added)

The report by Kendall does not elaborate on why "intentionally impure products" might be utilized or manufactured at DPG.[9]

A former member of the military disagrees with the purported "inadvertence" of the live anthrax mailing. Speaking under terms of confidentiality, a source with former military connections had this to say about the US's biological weapons program:

"...weaponizing bio & chem materials is in full swing at government research labs (Dugway & Tooele being one of the biggest – as I witnessed back in the late 1980s). The obvious thing is that they could not have shipped out such quantities with the level of relevant ease if they were not in full swing."

According to Department of Defense spokesperson, Adrian J.T. Rankine-Galloway, Major, U.S. Marine Corps, "To date, there have been no joint working groups in addition to the Republic of Korea-United States Biological Defense Cooperation Joint Working Group."

It would therefore appear that the other eight countries known to have received live anthrax from the US – Japan, United Kingdom, Australia, Canada, Italy, Germany, Norway and Switzerland – did not exhibit extensive concerns about the receipt of the active germ warfare agent.

--December 26, 2015

3

PANDEMIC WATCH: ANOTHER INSIDER ANNOUNCES THAT A GLOBAL PANDEMIC IS IMMINENT

D
r. J. Joseph Kim, founder and director of Inovio Pharmaceuticals, has recently declared that a global pandemic is "inevitable" in the next couple of years.

Quoted in an article in US News on December 24,[10] Dr. Kim opined that a global bird flu pandemic would result in a considerable death rate, stating, "I really believe we were lucky in 2009 [with the swine flu] because the strain that won out was not particularly lethal," he says. "Bird flu kills over 60 percent of people that it infects, regardless of health or age. It is a phenomenal killing machine – our only saving grace thus far is the virus has not yet jumped to humans."

Through his declaration of the imminent nature of a pandemic, Kim adds his name to a growing list of insiders who are stating that we are shortly facing a disease event of a global magnitude. WMD Center Executive Director Randall Larsen, former Senators Bob Graham and Jim Talent and Dr. Daniel Gerstein of the Department of Homeland Security have also been reported as making these predictions.

At the very time that our attention is focused on the possibility of losing our rights to defend ourselves via our potential loss of our second amendment rights, the insidious possibility of a global pandemic is lurking …. well, right under our pavement.

The possibility for utilization of the water system as a delivery system for a pandemic-type agent[11] remains salient. Recent disclosures as to the existence of impostor pharmaceuticals which may also induce disease and death, coupled with reams of documentation as to the dangers already resulting from vaccines, present a multiplicity of mechanisms for population reduction.

Truthfully, I prefer the word "genocide" to "population reduction." Given the selective nature of delivery systems already in place, it is very likely that when the (engineered) pandemic hits, it will only affect certain types of humans. It is not beyond the realm of possibility that at the time of deployment, our public health officials will declare that certain races "appeared" to be more vulnerable to the toxic agent, when in fact only predetermined groups were exposed. This is how selectivity in terms of delivery system works.*

Dr. J. Joseph Kim launched Inovio after working for Merck and Co, where he was a senior vaccine developer and led efforts in manufacturing and process development for several products and developmental therapeutics. These new products include vaccines for hepatitis as well as developmental vaccines and therapeutics for HIV/AIDS.

Merck has been under scrutiny for a number of years for problems with its products, including drugs such as Temodar, PegIntron, and Intron A. Questions have also been raised concerning the safety of some of Merck's vaccines. Some of the recent concerns follow:

- In 2008, the FDA issued a warning letter to the Merck vaccine production facility in Pennsylvania after citing multiple violations of manufacturing rules.

- In 2011, 13 vials of the Merck Gardasil vaccine, from six different countries were tested by SANE Vax, which found that all were contaminated with genetically modified HPV DNA. The package insert had claimed for the last five years that the vaccine contained no viral DNA.

- In 2011, Merck recalled over a million doses of HIB and HIB/Hep B vaccines due to possible contamination.

- Again in 2011, concerns were raised when Merck vaccines were found to be contaminated with plastic.

- Merck was again in the news in 2012 when headlines announced that its HIV vaccine actually appeared to facilitate the onset of the disease.

Dr. Kim left Merck and founded VGX Pharmaceuticals in 2000. He was appointed director and CEO of Inovio in 2009 and combined VGX with Inovio Biomedical in that year to form Inovio Pharmaceuticals.

Inovio continues to partner with Merck, according to the Inovio website.

Inovio is working on a universal flu vaccine and has also developed DNA vaccines which use the broken DNA of viruses rather than the viruses themselves. Inovio is also pioneering the use of electroporation in its vaccine delivery systems. This utilizes small pulses to open cell membranes for milliseconds, allowing strands of a virus's broken DNA to enter the cell.

Inovio has received $28 billion in funding over the past 24 months from the National Institutes of Health, most of which was allocated to the HIV vaccine, according to Dr. Kim. Inovio reports partnering with the Department of Homeland Security and the US military.

Dr. Kim is a member of The Global Agenda Council of the World Economic Forum.

Dr. Kim did not respond to calls from this reporter.

– January 7, 2013

---

* The Covid-19 agent is purportedly considerably more lethal for those of African descent. According to a CDC report released in June of 2020, blacks are far more likely to succumb to this virus than are whites.[12]

4

THINGS THAT GO BUMP IN THE NIGHT: KEEPING SKIPPY SAFE FROM THE TERR'ISTS

According to Randall Larsen, Executive Director of the WMD Center in Washington, DC, the terrorists' next target may be your peanuts.

Yep, Larsen is staying up at night with the worry beads due to the fact that all the nation's peanuts are processed at one plant, in North or South Carolina … he can't remember which. According to Larsen, the centralization of this facility provides an easy target for terrorists wielding chemical or biological weapons.

Larsen is a former Colonel in the United States Air Force and is a decorated Vietnam vet. He is a founding member of the WMD center, a not-for- profit research organization, along with former Senators Bob Graham (D-FL) and Jim Talent (R-MO). Larsen is also the national security advisor at the Center for Biosecurity, University of Pittsburgh Medical Center and is a senior fellow at the Homeland Security Policy institute at George Washington University.

In a recent telephone interview, Larsen opined that food terrorism is one the most significant threats faced by the nation.

Larsen also responded to questions about predictions being tendered concerning an imminent pandemic. "Pandemics," declared Larsen, "run in thirty-forty year cycles. We are overdue."

In fact, Larsen may have his numbers screwed up. The Spanish flu, which killed 20-40 million people worldwide, made its debut in 1918. The Asian flu killed about a million people in 1957-58 and only ten years later the Hong Kong flu killed just under a million.

Facts notwithstanding, the predictions persist that 2013 will be the Big One – either in terms of a terrorist attack or a pandemic. Not only have Larsen's colleagues, Talent and Graham, committed to this perception, but Dr. Daniel Gerstein of the Department of Homeland Security made just such a prediction last December at the Biological Weapons Convention, which took place in Geneva, Switzerland at the United Nations. "We expect a pandemic before the end of 2013," stated Gerstein.[13]

A Pandemic or A Biological Weapons Attack? Could They Be One and the Same?

Larsen pooh-poohed the idea that water systems might be a target for a domestic terrorist attack. He stated that, given the amount of pathogen necessary to contaminate a water system, it was highly unlikely that such an effort would be successful.

However, Larsen's perception is not shared by others in government nor by the scientific community. Last year, DHS chief Janet Napolitano issued a homeland security warning that dangerous terrorists had infiltrated utility companies and that the threat of an attack through infrastructure was emergent.

Her concerns were echoed just last week by Leon Panetta, who was reported as declaring that "are targeting the computer control systems that operate chemical, electricity and water plants, and those that guide transportation throughout the country." He went on to say that an aggressor nation or terrorist group could "could contaminate the water supply in major cities, or shut down the power grid across large parts of the country."[14]

The scientific community is also at odds with Larsen's assessment of the threat posed by a waterborne attack. A heavily footnoted report by the Congressional Research Service entitled "Terrorism and Security Issues Facing the Water Infrastructure Sector," stated that "Bioterrorism or chemical attacks could deliver widespread contamination with small amounts of microbiological agents or toxic chemicals, and could endanger the public health of thousands." (December 15, 2010)

During the course of our phone interview, this reporter suggested to Larsen that the danger posed by vulnerabilities inherent in the very configuration of water systems countrywide might present a compelling concern to those involved in protecting the United States from a terrorist attack. With his permission, this reporter forwarded a report detailing these vulnerabilities, which was submitted to the Critical Infrastructure unit of the Department of Homeland Security last August. The report is reproduced in its entirety, below.

> From: JANET PHELAN <janetcphelan@yahoo.com>
> Subject: Per our conversation today–vulnerability to bioterrorism through critical infrastructure
> To: nicc@dhs.gov
> Date: Friday, August 5, 2011, 3:42 PM

Ray,

I appreciate so much your speaking to me today at the Critical Infrastructure Command Center and taking my verbal report on my concerns as to critical vulnerabilities in the U.S. water systems, as currently configured. It is my understanding that work began sometime in the 1970s and that double lines were installed in cities across America. This has resulted in a critical vulnerability to insider attack through the water system. As you requested, I am sending you this email with links to articles on this subject.

As I stated in our call, which took place at approximately 5:45 pm ET on August 5, 2011, DHS Chief Janet Napolitano's concerns that terrorists may have infiltrated utility companies and may intend to launch an attack through water or other utilities may be well founded. In the articles below, you will see where I have interviewed a number of people working in pivotal positions in water systems and have found their responses to be specious and inaccurate. The false and misleading statements made by those named herein clearly attempt to redirect concern away from the very aspects of the water systems which provide the vulnerability to attack double lines and remote controlled valves, which are currently withholding what can potentially be released into the targeted households.

Here are the links to a number of articles I have authored concerning the possibility of bioterrorism in general and the potential use of the water system as a means of attacking selected portions of the U.S. populace. Some of these articles were published in hard copy newspapers and some were published on the Web. I cannot stress enough the selectivity provided by the system as currently configured.

I will look forward to hearing back from you shortly. I am currently out of the country and you may leave a message for me at 541 603-0514 or you may reach me by email.

Sincerely,
Janet Phelan
http://miami.indymedia.org/news/2007/05/8296.php
http://www.salem-news.com/articles/february242011/homeward-bound-jp.php
https://www.activistpost.com/2011/06/concerns-continue-to-mount-on-us.html
http://salem-news.com/articles/january282011/bioweapons-treaty-jp.php

Larsen's response was terse and to the point. On September 8, 2012, he sent me this message from his Iphone:

After reading some of your pieces on the Internet about the Patriot Act, I assure you we will have no further conversations or email exchanges. Sorry I wasted your time and mine.

Well, at least he has locked in on the Skippy terrorism. What a relief. I was beginning to think we might have a problem.

-- October 18, 2012

MIT States That Half of All Children May be Autistic by 2025 due to Monsanto

A senior scientist at MIT has declared that we are facing an epidemic of autism that may result in one half of all children being affected by autism in ten years.

Dr. Stephanie Seneff, who made these remarks during a panel presentation in Groton, MA last week, specifically cites the Monsanto herbicide, Roundup, as the culprit for the escalating incidence of autism and other neurological disorders. Roundup, which was introduced in the 1970's, contains the chemical glyphosate, which is the focal point for Seneff's concerns.

Roundup was originally restricted to use on weeds, as glyphosate kills plants. However, Roundup is now in regular use with crops. With the coming of GMOs, plants such as soy and corn were bioengineered to tolerate glyphosate, and its use dramatically increased. From 2001 to 2007, glyphosate use doubled, reaching 180 to 185 million pounds in the U.S. alone in 2007.

If you don't consume corn- on- the -cob or toasted soybeans, however, you are hardly exempt from the potential affects of consuming glyphosate. Wheat is now sprayed with Roundup right before it is harvested, making any consumption of non- organic wheat bread a sure source for the chemical. In addition, any products containing corn syrup, such as soft drinks, are also carrying a payload of glyphosate.

According to studies cited by Seneff, glyphosate engages "gut bacteria" in a process known as the shikimate pathway. This enables the chemical to interfere with the biochemistry of bacteria in our GI tract, resulting in the depletion of essential amino acids .

Monsanto has maintained that glyphosate is safe for human consumption, as humans do not have the shikimate pathway. Bacteria, however, does—including the flora that constitutes "gut bacteria."

It is this ability to affect gut bacteria that Seneff claims is the link which allows the chemical to get on board and wreak further damage. The connection between intestinal flora and neurological functioning is an ongoing topic of research. According to a number of studies, glyphosate depletes the amino acids tyrosine, tryptophan, and phenylalanine, which can then contribute to obesity, depression, autism, inflammatory bowel disease, Alzheimer's and Parkinson's.

Monsanto disagrees. The food and chemical giant has constructed a webpage with links to scientific studies pronouncing the safety of glyphosate.[15]

Other science writers have also taken up the Monsanto banner, scoffing at the scientific studies that prompted Seneff to make her claims. "They made it up!" pronounced Huffpost science writer Tamar Haspel, in an article thin on analysis but heavy on declarative prose.[16]

Others, such as Skeptoid writer and PhD physicist Eric Hall, take a more measured approach, and instead focus on the studies which prompted the glyphosate concerns. According to Hall, Seneff is making an error known as the "correlation/causation error," in which causality is inaccurately concluded when there exists only the fact that two separate items—in this case, the increased use of glyphosate and the increased incidence of autism—may be observed but are not, in fact, directly related.

Seneff's pronouncements focus specifically on the glyphosate issue. As we know, there are other potential tributaries which may be feeding the rise in autism and also causing age-related neurological conditions, such as Alzheimer's. These may include contents of vaccines, aluminum cooking ware as well as other potential sources for chemical consumption.

Some individuals, such as M.D. and radio host Rima Laibow have speculated on the intentionality behind this ostensible chemical siege against our gray matter. Laibow believes that the impetus may be to create an entire class of autistic individuals who will be suited only for certain types of work.

This harks back, eerily, to Aldous Huxley's classic *Brave New World*, in which individuals were pre-programmed from "conception" for eventual placement in one of five groups, designated as Alpha, Beta, and so on down to Epsilon, based on their programmed brain power. In Huxley's dystopian world, this class delineation by intellectual ability enabled society to function more smoothly.

Whatever may be driving the autistic/Alzheimer's diesel train, one thing is for certain: the spectre of half of our children coming into the world with significant brain damage constitutes a massive and undeniable wound to humanity. The rate of autism has skyrocketed from roughly one in every two thousand in the 1970's to the current rate of one in every sixty eight. Alzheimer's has become almost universal in the elderly. Seneff's predictions can only be ignored at grave risk to the human race.

--January 26, 2015

BAYER BUYS MONSANTO – MORE TO THIS MERGER THAN MEETS THE EYE

The chemical giant Bayer has just purchased the agricultural bio-technology company Monsanto for $66 billion. This union is redolent of marriages between members of medieval royalty, accomplished not out of love but out of a desire to keep the goods in the family while expanding the reach and control of the royals.

And in this case, the real nature of "the goods" requires special scrutiny. Monsanto is hardly an unknown quantity. The global company specializes in herbicides and genetically engineered seeds, most notably Roundup herbicide and the genetically modified Roundup Ready seed. The impact of Roundup has raised levels of alarm, as it is thought to contribute to the worldwide spike in autism, heart disease and other illnesses. Genetically engineered seeds have also engendered concerns and have been connected with an increased risk of certain types of cancer.[17]

Bayer is a global German-based behemoth, producing both chemicals and pharmaceuticals. Unknown to many, however, is that its reach extends into water, as well.

Like food, even perhaps surpassing food, water is also life. Bayer was founded in 1863 and later became part of IG Farben, which manufactured Zyklon B used to gas Jews, Gypsies, political dissidents, homosexuals and others during the Hitler years. Following the war, IG Farben was broken up into a number of smaller companies, including AGFA, BASF, Sanofi and Bayer.

Through fluoridating the water in the concentration camps, the Nazis maintained a level of chemical control over those imbibing the water. It is the contention of this author, based on years of research, that plans exist within the United States and her allies to potentially use domestic water systems as delivery systems for a chemical or bioweapons attack under the guise of a naturally occurring pandemic. As extreme as these contentions may be, the supporting documentation is overwhelming, including blueprints, changes in domestic bioweapons legislation which grant immunity to government agents for violating the existing biological weapons laws, changes in legislation to criminalize government officers for revealing information about water systems and more.[18]

On the surface, Bayer's involvement with water may seem peripheral. Bayer's website states a concern for water-use efficiency and sustainability and admits only that "Bayer operates production facilities around the world, but only 2% of its water usage takes place in areas officially classified by the World Resources Institute as water scarce."

What sounds like a fairly modest reach into water is belied by the other corporate positions held by its governing and supervisory board members. Marijn Dekkers was CEO for Bayer from October 2010 until April 30, 2016. During this period he also sat on the Board for General Electric, which is also heavily invested in water technologies.[19] The chairman of the Board of Management at Bayer from April 2002 until September 30, 2010, Werner Wenning, is also a member of the Supervisory Board of Siemens AG, München. From May 2011 to June 2016, he was also Chairman of the Supervisory Board of E.ON AG, Düsseldorf.

Both Siemens and E.ON are heavily into water. Siemens reports that "(it) offers a comprehensive portfolio of integrated automation solutions and drives for water and wastewater treatment, seawater desalination, as well as solutions for water network and pipeline management."

E.ON Energie's principal water-related activities are centered in the German stock exchange-listed company Gelsenwasser AG ("Gelsenwasser") According to the SEC, "Gelsenwasser is the largest privately held water utility in Germany (based on volume of water deliveries)."[20]

The former top dog at Bayer also maintained a significant involvement with water companies. Dr. Manfred Schneider, who was Chairman of Bayer from 2002-2012 was also Chairman of the Board for the utility giant, RWE. RWE, through a subsidiary named American Water Works, was quietly buying up water systems throughout the United States.[21]

Bayer's involvement with water does not end with its Chairmen, however. Other individuals sitting on the supervisory and management boards of Bayer have extensive involvement in other corporations that treat and deliver water. These corporations include Lonza, Emerson, Linde, Evonik, Innovationsregion Rheinisches Revier GmbH, Cabot Corporation, Envia Mitteldeutsche Energie AG and Sulzer, to name a few. Names of individuals who sit on the Bayer boards and have other corporate involvements with water companies include Sue Rataj, Petra Reinbold-Knape, Thomas Ebbeling, Dr. Clemens Börsig and Dr. Klaus Sturany, among others.

Werner Baumann was appointed Chairman of the Board at Bayer in May of this year and appears to have no other corporate ties.

The marriage of Monsanto and Bayer may well result in a consolidation of control over not only the food we eat and the medicine we take, but also the very water we drink. These three consumables — food, medicine and water — constitute the very stuff of life. If ever there was a corporate behemoth positioned to significantly affect our future, this may be it.

--September 30, 2016

PORTON DOWN'S LEGACY OF DEATH: INQUEST TO TAKE PLACE SHORTLY CONCERNING DEATH OF SCIENTIST

In April of 2012, Dr. Richard Holmes took a stroll in the woods in Wiltshire, England. His body was found two days later.

Holmes is one of several Porton Down scientists who have died under questionable circumstances. The death in November 2001 of Vladimir Pasechnik was ruled to be a stroke, although co-workers stated that Pasechnik was in good health. Vladimir Pasechnik was a Russian defector who first alerted the West to the extensive clandestine research into biological warfare taking place within the Soviet Union.

His death was, oddly, belatedly announced by Dr. Christopher Davis of Virginia. Davis was the member of British intelligence who debriefed Dr. Pasechnik at the time of his defection. The announcement of Pasechnik's death did not come in England until a month after he died. Interestingly, Pasechnik was also debriefed by a Dr. David Kelly, head of microbiology at Porton Down, which is England's top secret chemical, biological and nuclear laboratory.

Dr. David Kelly, whose body was also found in the woods, had been invited to take the position of chief microbiologist at Porton Down in 1986. Later, he worked extensively with Dr. Wouter Basson of South Africa's clandestine Project Coast. Basson was known to be working on a "black's only" bioweapon. When South Africa's apartheid government fell, Basson was subsequently charged with an assortment of crimes, including murder. He skated on all the charges and is now a successful cardiologist in Durbanville, South Africa.

Another scientist who collaborated with Kelly and Basson, Dr. Larry Ford of Irvine, California died in 2001 of a shotgun blast that was ruled a suicide. Police found guns, ammunition and explosives when they dug up his yard. Cholera, botulinum, salmonella and typhoid were also located in vials in his refrigerator. All told, 266 bottles and vials of lethal toxins were found in the Ford home.

The CIA declined to comment on Ford's intelligence connections.

Dr. Kelly's death in 2004—in the same woods that were to later claim the body of Dr. Richard Holmes—sent shock waves through the clandestine scientific community. Kelly reportedly died after slashing his wrists and consuming a cocktail of painkillers. His death was subsequently ruled a suicide.

However, according to the publication the Daily Mail, thirteen respected doctors declared that it was medically impossible for Dr. Kelly to have died in this manner.[22]

Andrew Gilligan, a reporter for BBC, claimed that Kelly had recently given him and other reporters information that proved the government had exaggerated the Iraqi danger in its "dossier" in order to justify the war against Iraq. Kelly was also reported to be writing a "tell-all" book.

The *Daily Mail* also reported that "at 8 AM, half an hour before Dr. Kelly's body was discovered under the tree, three officers in dark suits from MI5's Technical Assessment Unit were at his house. The computers and the hard-disk containing the 40,000 words of the explosive book were carried away. They have never been seen since."

In 2004, Kelly's replacement as the chief scientist for chemical and biological defence at the Ministry of Defence's laboratory at Porton Down, Dr. Paul Norman, died when the plane he was piloting crashed near Devon.

The Wiltshire coroner's office stated this week that Dr. Holmes' coroner's inquest will take place shortly. Dr. Holmes had recently left his employment at Porton Down before his fateful walk in the woods. It is unclear why he resigned. Within a month after leaving Porton Down, he was dead.

-- May 18, 2013

8

LAWSUIT SEEKS INJUNCTION AGAINST EPA "GAS CHAMBER" EXPERIMENTS

A lawsuit filed in federal court in Alexandria, Virginia seeks injunctive relief from human experimentation being conducted by the Environmental Protection Agency. The experiments involve gassing human subjects with PM2.5.

The New York Health Department defines PM2.5 as follows: "Fine particulate matter (PM2.5) is an air pollutant that is a concern for people's health when levels in air are high."

In one of these experiments, individuals were given a breathing apparatus through which they inhaled diesel fuel piped in from a truck parked outside.

The lawsuit cites the EPA's own determination on the dangers posed by PM2.5: "In the Agency's most recent scientific assessment of PM2.5., the EPA concluded that PM2.5 can kill people shortly after exposure." The suit goes on to state that "EPA's 2004 and 2009 scientific assessment expressly found that there is no safe level of PM2.5."

The lawsuit, filed by American Tradition Institute Environmental Law Center, states that these experiments have been conducted at the University of North Carolina and have been ongoing since 2004. The suit names both the EPA and its Administrator Lisa Jackson as plaintiffs.

In its answer to the suit, the EPA admits that PM2.5 may pose a health risk but states that the overall public benefit outweighs the risk to individual subjects. In addition, the EPA's response to the request for the restraining order states:

> While small risks to individuals may evidence themselves as much larger overall public health risks when large populations are exposed to ambient levels of PM2.5 , this does not change the fact that the risk for individuals that do not exhibit these health conditions will be small.

The suit alleges that the subjects were not informed of the dangers of inhaling PM2.5, a contention which the EPA denies.

The EPA's response to the suit also states that the court lacks jurisdiction to hear this case.

In a recent interview, the counsel for plaintiffs, Dr. David Schnare announced "The EPA has lost its way." Schnare, who worked for three decades for the EPA, first as a scientist and policy analyst and later as an attorney, denounced the experiments as "illegal," and stated: "They imposed risks without telling people."

– November 27, 2012

STATE OF THE SCIENCE

9

The Strange Convergence of Technologies of Life and of Extermination

The peculiar convergence of technologies which seem on the surface to stand in opposition to each other may, in fact, be working towards a common goal of reinventing life as we know it.

What we are referring to here are technologies which seem to be in the service of creating life and those which are directly implicated in ending life.

On the one hand, we see, as in the recent reports of successful artificial manufacture of a rodent embryo, where science is increasingly leveraging towards breaking the God Barrier, in its attempts to create life from non-life.[1] This subtrend, (or is it a primary impetus?) in the life sciences took a major stride forward when the human genome was sequenced back around the turn of the new millennium.[2]

Articles now proliferate on genetic sequencing of diseases as well as on the emerging technologies of gene editing. With the advent of genetic editing tools, such as CRISPR Cas9, the ability of science to reconfigure life, to alter its basic code, became a reality. Even in the face of recent publications stating that CRISPR Cas9 is not the precise tool it was first thought to be, and is in fact more like an axe or shredder than a scalpel, science's infatuation with gene editing marches on.

However, alongside the impetus to create life we also see a steady acceleration in technologies of death. Mass death. Nowhere in the proliferation of weapons systems is this convergence of technologies more salient than in the existence of gene weapons. Despite protestations by the military that such weapons do not exist, reports detail their deployment against both groups and individuals.[3]

Numerous publications are now reporting that the ubiquitous emanations from WiFi and cell phones and other electromagnetics cause cancer and brain damage. The proliferation of concerns of the harmful effects of 5G only scratch the surface. A new wave of researchers, such as physicist Dr. Katherine Horton, are claiming that electromagnetics have been weaponized and are being deployed against selected US citizens. Horton declares that the deployment of these weapons has far surpassed the testing stage and that these weapons are now being levied for the purpose of "slow kill."[4]

Scientists have recently decried the development of autonomous robot killers. As reported widely, over 2400 scientists recently signed a statement declaring that they will not participate in the development or manufacture of robots that can identify and attack people without human oversight.[5] No, this is not a science fiction novel or a dystopian "Terminator" fantasy. The technology involved in producing drone killer robots has advanced to the point where Britain, in a telling display of doublespeak, has unveiled its plan to build a pilotless military aircraft at the same point that it insists it will not fund autonomous lethal weapons.

And the US military is already in R and D mode concerning linking soldiers' brains to a computer interface.[6]

Ostensibly the UN would be the logical locus for international agreements concerning lethal weapons systems. The UN, however, appears to be operating deceptively in this regard. When documents were turned over the Biological Weapons Convention in Geneva concerning the fact that the US had put into place a covert delivery system for biological and chemical weapons delivery,[7] the UN retaliated.

ITHACA is the NGO which lodged this report with the BWC at the UN. The UN subsequently falsely reported in its documents that ITHACA was a mental institution. When Daniel Feakes, with the Biological Weapons Convention Implementation Support Unit was contacted with questions as to who inserted this bizarre information into the official UN report, Feakes refused to answer.

The fact that international agreements concerning biological warfare as well as chemical warfare are being subverted by internal legislation in the US increases the concern that these technologies of death are being developed and readied for use. The US maintains domestic legislation which permits her to use these weapons, flying in the face of the mandates of the accords.[8] While the chemical and biological weapons treaties specifically state that the member nations are pledged not to develop these weapons and are to pass legislation banning these weapons, the US continues to quietly and without fanfare thumb her nose at the treaty mandates.

In her widely acclaimed dystopian sci fi trilogy, *The Year of the Flood*, author Margaret Atwood posits a future in which a rogue and psychologically disturbed scientist is able to wipe out nearly all human life while substituting a new version of humanity, in which he has bred out certain characteristics which he felt to be problematic and contributing to humanity's perennial struggles with war, egotism and sex. In Atwood's trilogy, The Big Kill was indeed accomplished through a covert chem/bio attack. When one views the reality of science's efforts in the direction of reconfiguring the genetic code and creating a whole new strain of humans, at the very time that mass death technologies are being put into play, one wonders if Atwood's books were fiction or prophesy.

The only difference between the scenario advanced in her trilogy and the one which appears to be developing before our very eyes would be that, by making a frankly pathological scientist the sole perpetrator, Atwood's vision excluded the collusion between innumerable corporate, government and scientific entities, a collusion which is both far reaching and far too entrenched.

July 27, 2018

10

GENE EDITING:
THE DUAL-USE CONUNDRUM

D ual-use may be best understood by considering the functions of a knife. Used against an enemy, a knife can be deadly. In the hands of a skilled surgeon, a knife may be life-saving, removing a gangrenous appendage or excising a cancerous mass.

Wikipedia defines dual-use this way: "In politics and diplomacy, dual-use is technology that can be used for both peaceful and military aims. More generally speaking, dual-use can also refer to any technology which can satisfy more than one goal at any given time."

Behind the debate over the Iran nuclear deal lurked the dual-use issue. On the one hand, there were those claiming that Iran had every right to develop nuclear power in pursuit of peaceful aims. In the other camp were those who maintained that possession of nuclear technology was a path towards developing nuclear weapons, and in the hands of a regime hostile to America's purported friend and ally, Israel, was too dangerous to be allowed to manifest.

Dual-use has implications reaching beyond nuclear science. Those watching the development of what is termed "biodefense" are uncomfortably aware that the production of countermeasures for biological weapons also necessitates the development and possession of the weapon itself. Increasingly, accusations are being levied that countermeasure research may be a "cover" for weapons development.

In the biological sciences, the debate concerning dual-use technology just ramped up a notch. Recently, the office of the US Director of National Intelligence issued a report declaring that genome editing constituted a "weapon of mass destruction." Stated the report: "Given the broad distribution, low cost, and accelerated pace of development of this dual-use technology, its deliberate or unintentional misuse might lead to far-reaching economic and national security implications."

Although the report did not cite Crispr-Cas9 by name, the reference to this gene editing tool was clear. The Crispr-Cas9 was developed in 2012 by Jennifer Doudna, a Berkeley professor of biochemistry and molecular biology and is considered revolutionary in its potential impact on life sciences. Cheap (one can acquire the components for $60 online) and easy to use, the Crisp-Cas9 allows scientists to edit genes in order to correct genetic illnesses.[9]

Doudna's discovery has some folks positively chirping. Gushes Techcrunch,

> "Doudna found a protein in Streptococcus bacteria that will "snip" certain DNA at precise areas. It's like a sort of biological scissors that cuts the DNA where you want to cut. And it has the potential to eradicate cancer, Parkinson's, herpes, or even do away with disease-bearing mosquitoes. It can also make microorganisms produce spider silk, the scent of roses, glow in the dark and many other actions so far. What Doudna has embarked upon, in short, is the find of the century."[10]

Applied to the human germline, however, some darker concerns emerge. "Germline editing" would impact those cells which would transmit the alterations to future generations. And it is this potential that has Director of National Intelligence James Clapper worried.

For not only can the Crispr-Cas9 replace cells which are causing illness; it can also be used in editing heritable cells in embryos which will pass on the changes. It is now possible for scientists (and whomever else has the 60 bucks) to create a new "line" of human beings. And here potentially lies the dual-use conundrum of Crispr-Cas9.

The office of the DNI declined to comment further on the inclusion of germline editing as a potential "weapon of mass destruction." However, the DNI report contains some language that deserves further scrutiny and elucidates why this technology has hit the intelligence community's radar.

According to the DNI report:

> "Research in genome editing conducted by countries with different regulatory or ethical standards than those of Western countries probably increases the risk of the creation of potentially harmful biological agents or products."[11]

The regulatory standards of Western countries, however, do not necessarily prohibit this kind of research.

While Great Britain is often cited as having laws which prohibit germline editing, the British government permits, at its discretion, this research. Recently, TIME Magazine reported that Great Britain has given the green light to a germline editing research project. According to TIME, "The U.K.'s Human Fertilization and Embryo Authority (HFEA) decided to approve a researcher's request to use Crispr to permanently change DNA in a human embryo."[12]

The project, which is launched by the Francis Crick Institute, is specifically a research-only project, we are told. "I promise you she has no intention of the embryos ever being put back into a woman for development," Robin Lovell-Badge, group leader at the Crick Institute, told TIME."

Germline editing got a big dose of publicity last year, when it was reported that researchers in China had accomplished germline editing on embryos, also without implanting the embryos. As a result, an international summit was called last December, for the purposes of examining the ethics of this technology. The summit, which took place in Washington, DC, issued a statement which fell short of condemning this research. Instead, the summit asserted that the technical and ethical issues should be settled before anyone attempts to edit the human germline.

The closing statement read:

> "It would be irresponsible to proceed with any clinical use of germline editing unless and until the relevant safety and efficacy issues have been resolved, based on appropriate understanding and balancing of risks, potential benefits, and alternatives, and there is broad societal consensus about the appropriateness of the proposed application."[13]

The US does not prohibit the use of germline editing. The National Institutes of Health has declared, "NIH will not fund any use of gene-editing technologies in human embryos. The concept of altering the human germline in embryos for clinical purposes has been debated over many years from many different perspectives, and has been viewed almost universally as a line that should not be crossed."

While appearing to condemn the use of this technology, what the NIH has done here is to allow it to be privately funded. This opens the door for wealthy eugenicists, such as Bill Gates, to create an entirely new strain of human beings, and to do so without violating any law.

This may be seen as an aspect of a duality in US law, which appears to discourage while actually is encouraging certain types of activity.

The fix may be in. Recently, the Hastings Center announced it received a grant to study the ethics of human genome editing. In its news release,

Hastings stated that "The three-year project, which is supported with nearly $1 million from the Templeton Foundation, is examining a variety of fundamental questions about how use of gene editing in humans might affect 'human flourishing' and core human values such as love, compassion, acceptance, and respect for those with disability."

The Templeton Foundation funds research into eclectic areas and provides grant money to speculative research on spiritual issues. Sir John Templeton was a follower of the Chicago School neoliberal giant, Milton Friedman, whose ideas translated into dollar signs for the well-to-do and a short stick for anyone else. Along with funding research into "goodness" and "moral character," the Foundation has provided donations to the neoconservative think tank, the Cato Institute, and has funded research into GMOs.

At least one of the principal researchers in the Hastings Center genome research project may have her mind already made up. Addressing the argument that parents will want to use this new technology to provide their children with a better prospective future, Hastings's research director Josephine Johnston wrote: "It will be difficult to ban the use of gene editing for this purpose, because doing so would restrict both parental rights and reproductive freedom."

Erik Parens, who is also one of the chief researchers in this project, has already been found leaning towards a future which involves genetically modified humans. In an article entitled, "Can Parents Be Trusted with Gene Editing Technology?" Parens discusses the obligation of parents to not only accept their children, but to shape them. Parens writes, "Grasping the nature of this tension in the context of embryo editing forces us to revisit the question, 'Is eugenics inherently bad?' It forces us to see why it won't be enough to assert, 'You can't do that, it's eugenics!' — and why we need to distinguish between good and bad eugenic practices."[14]

There is some essential hubris involved in the very concept of this level of tinkering with nature. Gene drives, defined by Science Magazine as "… stimulating biased inheritance of particular genes to alter entire populations of organisms," have got some thinking about the potential for eradicating entire populations. MIT's Sculpting Evolution recently waxed rhapsodic about these possibilities:

> "Gene drives could benefit human health by altering insect populations that currently spread diseases such as malaria, schistosomiasis, dengue, and Lyme so that they can no longer transmit

the disease to humans. They could improve the sustainability of agriculture by reducing the need for and toxicity of pesticides and herbicides. Finally, they could aid ecological restoration by removing invasive species and bolstering the defenses of threatened organisms. Collectively, they offer a way to solve biological problems with biology instead of broadly toxic pesticides and bulldozers. On a metaphorical level, we are finally learning to speak with the living world using nature's own language."[15]

Through the centuries, the potential of remaking the world in a "better" image has motivated both political activists and mad dictators, Gandhis and Hitlers. Before the final weighing in on dual-use technologies such as genome editing, it might be best to revisit the dual nature of humanity and how power tends to corrupt whomever bears its mantle.

July 11, 2016

11

Genetic Weapons—
Can Your DNA Kill You?

It is a scene out of a futuristic political thriller—the Secretary of State issues secret orders for embassy officials to collect the DNA of foreign heads of state while the President, speaking at a $1000 a plate dinner, is surrounded by a contingent of Secret Service agents wiping clean his drinking glasses and picking up stray hair follicles. They are not just protecting the President—they are protecting the President's DNA.

If this sounds like a script treatment for a Hollywood version of a Philip K. Dick novel, consider this: The Secretary of State's name is Hillary Clinton and her directives to embassies were uncovered in a 2010 WikiLeaks cable release. The President in this scenario is Barack Obama and the Secret Service unit pledged to protect his DNA is a group of Navy stewards, as revealed in the 2009 book by Ronald Kessler, titled *In the President's Secret Service.*

Our government's DNA obsession was again in the news this week as the Supreme Court handed down a decision, worthy of penning by George Orwell, that law enforcement collection of arrestees' DNA is not an invasion of privacy. The decision likened DNA to fingerprints, neatly sidestepping the fact that a person's complete genetic makeup is contained in those drops of blood that the police can now collect with impunity and without fear of a civil rights lawsuit.

Beyond the obvious surface concerns that this decision violates both the Fourth Amendment and the subsequent exclusionary rule, there are further, deeper concerns as to why our government is so keen on collecting our DNA.[16]

The stated aim of furthering crime solution sounds a bit tinny when one realizes that the government is also collecting the DNA of newborns. President Bush signed The Newborn Screening Saves Lives Act of 2007, which formally codified the process that the federal government has been engaged in for years, screening the DNA of all newborn babies in the U.S.[17]

Since we are not yet threatened with the spectre of toddlers robbing banks or committing rape, one must look further to discern what is the big deal about our DNA.

Back in 1997, Dr. Wayne Nathanson warned a meeting of the Science and Ethics Department of the Medical Society of the United Kingdom that "gene therapy" might be turned to insidious uses and result in "gene weapons," which could be used to target specific people containing a specific genetic structure. These weapons, Nathanson warned, "could be delivered not only in the forms already seen in warfare such as gas and aerosol, but could also be added to water supplies, causing not only death but sterility and birth defects in targeted groups."[18]

Decades before Dr. Nathanson's highly publicized warning, the U.S. Government was already hard at work in scientific endeavors to find gene and ethnic specific weapons. In an article entitled "Ethnic Weapons," published in the Military Review in 1970, the author, Dr. Carl A. Larson, was found rhapsodizing about the state of technology facilitating the targeting of ethnic groups with covert weapons. Wrote Larson: "Surrounded with clouds of secrecy, a systematic search for new incapacitating agents is going on in many laboratories. The general idea, as discussed in open literature, was originally that of minimum destruction."

However, his tone soon changes and he writes, somewhat chillingly, that "It is quite possible to use incapacitating agents over the entire range of offensive operations, from covert activities to mass destruction."

Larson concludes with the following stark declaration: "The enzymatic process for RNA production has been known for some years but now the factors have been revealed which regulate the initiation and specificity of enzyme production. Not only have the factors been found, but their inhibitors. Thus, the functions of life lie bare to attack."

Dr. Wouter Basson's research for Project Coast, the biological and chemical warfare unit under the apartheid government in South Africa, was known to be focused on developing a "blacks only" bioweapon. Basson, who was tied to intelligence facilities and labs in both Great Britain and the U.S., has been reported to have been successful in his endeavors, which were taking place back in the seventies. According to sources close to Basson, his research entailed locating substances which would attach onto melanin. Melanin is present in high degrees in darker colored skin.

Since Basson's work on this project, the rates of hypertension and diabetes have skyrocketed in people of color—specifically those of African descent and also indigenous, brown skinned populations. In some communities, the incidence of these diseases is now reported as up to 50%. Consonant with the reports that this disease-producing melanin-related substance has been leaked into processed food, one finds the spiking rates of the "silent killers," hypertension and diabetes, to be present in the developed world, where people eat more processed food. In rural Africa, for example, where the population eats food from natural sources, the rates of diabetes and hypertension have remained constant over the years.

The mapping of the human genome satisfied the requisites for creating gene specific weapons. Geneticists have maintained that developing an ethnic weapon is actually far more difficult than creating a gene weapon to target a specific person. The differences between groups are apparently much smaller than the differences between individuals and therefore the creation of a genetic weapon to target, for example, a head of state or a President is far less challenging than creating such a weapon to target an entire race.

The FBI admits to a database of around 13 million offenders, many only arrested and never charged with a crime. According to Twila Brase, President of Citizens Council for Health Freedom, around 4 million samples (filed with the babies' names) are collected each year by State Health Departments. Some states, such as Minnesota, have been collecting newborn DNA samples since the mid-eighties. Minnesota alone is reported to have a newborn database of over 1.5 million samples.

The delivery systems for a DNA weapon would be easy: Everything.

Because the weaponized genetic material would only affect the target, the weapon could be leaked into the food supply, the water supply or sprayed in an airborne delivery system, such as the inexplicable chemtrails that are now blanketing our skies. And should a low profile target suddenly die, who would ever know that he died of a gene based weapon? Should the target be high profile, like perhaps a Hugo Chavez or Canada's Jack Layton, who would be able to trace a deadly disease back to a weapon targeting his DNA?

The insistence of the U.S. Government that it is only trying to protect its citizens from a terrorist threat is the tried and true cover of plausible deniability. Under the mantle of "protection," our rights have been systematically stripped away while wars abroad have been launched against the Semitic peoples of the Middle East. Genetic based weapons are another tool in the plausible deniability eugenics tool box. They may, in fact, be one of the most powerful tools.

--June 9, 2013

12

DOCTOR WHO RAN BIOWARFARE UNIT FACES SENTENCING

D r. Wouter Basson, who headed up Project Coast, the biological and chemical warfare unit under South Africa's apartheid government in the 1980s, will face sentencing by the Health Professions Council of South Africa on June 5.

Basson (dubbed "Dr. Death" by the South African media) was found guilty in December of 2013 of charges that he "acted unprofessionally" in manufacturing and supplying poisonous substances to security forces during the apartheid era.

Basson was previously charged at the Truth and Reconciliation Hearings that took place in South Africa following the dissolution of the apartheid government. In 1999, he faced charges in Pretoria High Court for murder and fraud, among a total of 67 charges, for allegedly overseeing plans to poison Namibian fighters with muscle relaxants, to infect water with cholera, and to deliver a baboon foetus to intimidate Nobel Peace Prize winner archbishop emeritus Desmond Tutu. His trial lasted two years and over 200 witnesses testified against him. He was the sole witness in his defense, in which he declared that everything he did, he did as a soldier.

He was acquitted. Basson currently is a successful cardiologist in Cape Town.

Much of what Basson actually accomplished is still a secret. He was known to have been engaged in genetic research and to be developing a blacks-only bioweapon.

There is evidence that Basson was successful in this endeavor. According to a scientist who worked alongside Basson under the apartheid government, this blacks-only bioweapon was to attach onto melanin (darker skinned people have more melanin in their skin). Citing his security agreement with the government, the scientist agreed to speak under conditions of anonymity, and stated he believed that Basson did in fact create this weapon.

Other sources indicate that this bioweapon was deployed on a grand scale, having been leaked into processed food. A confidential source in US intelligence stated that the spiking epidemic of the "silent killers" of hypertension and diabetes in people of color is due to the success of Basson's research and subsequent deployment of a genetic weapon which attaches onto melanin and was leaked into the food supply.

The incidence of diabetes and hypertension in people of color has indeed skyrocketed since Basson's days with Project Coast. According to the National Minority Organ Tissue Transplant Education Program (MOTTEP), 25% of African Americans between the ages of 65-75 have diabetes. The prevalence in women appears to even higher, with MOTTEP reporting that 25% of African American women over the age of 55 are afflicted with diabetes.

Hypertension is reported as most prevalent in the African American population. It affects about one out of every three African Americans, as opposed to one in five for the population at large. Complications of hypertension include heart attack, stroke, kidney failure, and blindness.

Looking at another group with high melanin content in skin, MOTTEP reports that the rates of diabetes among native Americans are the highest in the world, with over 12% in those over 19 years of age. Also reporting high are Latino-Americans, with 24% of Mexican Americans within the US and 26% of Puerto Ricans with diabetes.

According to the International Journal of Diabetes in Developing Countries, "from 1959 to the mid-1980s, medical statistics showed that the prevalence rate of diabetes in Africa was equal to or less then 1.4%, with the exception of South Africa, where the rate was estimated to be as high as 3.6% in 2001. But, by 1994, the continent-wide prevalence of diabetes mellitus stood at 3 million and was then predicted to double or triple by the year 2010." In fact, the prevalence has more than tripled. According to the International Diabetes Foundation (IDF), the 2010 numbers for those afflicted with diabetes in Africa have exceeded 12 million.[19] Peculiarly, the WHO continues to report low prevalence in Africa.

Supporting a hypothesis of food-related increase in prevalence, the International Diabetes Foundation reports that: "The highest prevalences are among the ethnic Indian population of Tanzania and South Africa. There is also a marked urban/rural difference in diabetes prevalence, with consequent likely increases as more people move to urban areas." Those in urban areas would be more dependent, of course, on processed food.

According to the IDF, "it is estimated that at least 1 in 20 deaths of those aged 20 to 79 years is due to diabetes. "

The food connection was also reported by the Voice of America, although the emphasis was given to portion size rather than content.[20] VOA reports:

> "Paul Madden, Project Hope's senior advisor for non-communicable diseases, explained that diabetes is rapidly spreading throughout sub-Saharan Africa, and even other developing countries around the world, largely due to lifestyle changes. People generally are not as active as previous generations, and they are in jobs that require them to sit or stand for long periods of time. Another reason for the increase in the rate of diabetes is eating processed food.
>
> "The way things are packaged, they're often in bigger portion sizes than the body needs. So it's the portion sizes, lack of activity. In some of the villages and towns and cities in Africa, it's people are living longer, and as you live longer and get less active, and also taking in a few too many calories on some days, and if you do that over many years, you gain weight," explained Madden.

No kidding...

But is it the "Coca-Cola syndrome"– that is, the increased sugar intake by those consuming processed foods – that has resulted in the diabetes epidemic or is it something else?

Back to our Dr. Basson. In a chilling admission by Dr. Basson, made during an interview with New York filmmaker Rob Coen several years ago, Basson crowed that developing the blacks-only bioweapon was "the most fun I ever had."[21] Elsewhere in the video clip, Basson refuses to answer questions having to do with his relationship with US and British intelligence, connections which involved the now deceased Dr. David Kelly and trips to Langley.[22]

At one point in the video, there is an effort to explain Basson's bizarre admission as possibly pertaining to work involved with sterilization. That work, however, could not be considered a genetic weapon and may be evidence of further attempts to obscure the exact nature of Basson's work and its reach.

One thing is for sure. Dr. Wouter Basson appears to be tightly wrapped in teflon. His sentencing by the medical board this coming week will entail a possible fine, medical license suspension or probation. Whether his work as "Dr. Death" involved not only the murders of regime-unfriendly people years ago, but also involved a trajectory into the present health crisis among people of color, worldwide, is a question that Basson apparently won't be answering.

--June 3, 2013

Update from Wikipedia: *"On 18 December 2013, the HPCSA found Basson guilty of unprofessional conduct on four charges. On 4 June 2014 sentencing procedure was postponed due to unavailability of counsel.*

On 27 March 2019, six years after Basson was found guilty of unethical conduct by an HPCSA committee, the Gauteng High Court ruled that there was bias on the part of the committee members that presided over the disciplinary hearing. The judge ruled that the proceedings (instituted by the HPCSA against Basson) were irregular and unfair and illustrated a total disregard for the rights of Basson. The hearing (and, therefore, the finding of unethical conduct by the committee) was accordingly set aside."

13

First GMO Corn, then Frankenfish, and Now — Get Ready for Designer Babies

We knew it was coming to this. The GMO revolution wasn't going to stop at our dinner table. But did we think it would happen so soon?

The first week in December, delegates from the top three gene-editing countries—China, the UK and the US—met in Washington, DC for a symposium on the future of gene-editing. For those not familiar with the parlance, gene editing refers to the ability to alter the DNA of an embryo in a manner which affects the germline. The germline is defined as follows: "In biology and genetics, the germline in a multicellular organism is that population of its bodily cells that are so differentiated or segregated that in the usual processes of reproduction they may pass on their genetic material to the progeny."

In other words, what happens to the germline will affect the offspring and subsequent generations.

The possibilities inherent in such manipulation are staggering. Not only could genetic diseases be removed from the developing embryo, but new and better attributes could be factored in. Mankind could face the possibility that crippling genetic diseases, such as Tay-Sachs or Huntington's Disease could be forever banished, while a brave new crop of humans, with enhanced intellectual abilities or enhanced musculature, for example, could be harvested.

The symposium was convened with some urgency after the disclosure that researchers in China had reported this past April that they had launched the first attempt to edit the DNA of human embryos. The Chinese project was undertaken to correct a rare and often fatal blood disorder, called beta thalassemia. China's effort was followed by an application, made in September, by a British research group to edit human embryos for research purposes.

Behind all this gene editing lies a new technology, which works like the "find and replace" function on a word processor. The most popular in this new buffet of tools is the Crispr-Cas9, which was invented by Dr. Jennifer Doudna. Dr. Doudna is a Professor of Chemistry and of Molecular and Cell Biology at the University of California, Berkeley and has also been an investigator with the Howard Hughes Medical Institute since 1997. The Crispr-Cas9 works in the following manner—first it locates the gene to be edited, then makes the desired alteration, either by deleting it or fixing it. Doudna has virtually revolutionized medicine with her invention, which is reportedly simple to use.

The symposium was expected to produce a call for a moratorium on this research, while the ethical implications could be sorted out. Surprisingly, that is not what eventuated. The final formal statement by the International Summit on Human Gene Editing Organizing Committee in fact left the door open.[23]

The Committee, which is comprised of ten scientists and two bioethicists, called on the "Big Three" in gene editing to take charge:

> "We therefore call upon the national academies that co-hosted the summit – the U.S. National Academy of Sciences and U.S. National Academy of Medicine; the Royal Society; and the Chinese Academy of Sciences – to take the lead in creating an ongoing international forum to discuss potential clinical uses of gene editing; help inform decisions by national policymakers and others; formulate recommendations and guidelines; and promote coordination among nations."

In a non-binding recommendation, the Committee also called for the inhibition of gene editing on viable embryos, stating "if in the process of research, early human embryos or germline cells undergo gene editing, the modified cells should not be used to establish a pregnancy."

The three day conference, which was attended by science heavyweights (as well as by some family members with sick children), resulted in an airing of some of the issues surrounding this new science.

Harvard's George Church made a presentation which propounded a viewpoint that challenged concerns about the fall-out from gene editing.

Dr. Church, who is a Professor of Genetics at Harvard Medical School, has written articles supporting germline editing and diminishing the possible repercussions. In a recent article in Nature, he wrote,

> "Human-germline editing is not special with respect to permanence or consent. Replacing deleterious versions of genes with

common ones is unlikely to lead to unforeseen effects and is probably reversible. Even if the editing was difficult to reverse, this would not be especially unsafe compared with other commonly inherited risks."[24]

In 2005, Church launched a project called the Personal Genome Project. In this effort, which is billed as "the world's only open-access information on human genomic, environmental & trait data," individuals are recruited to have their own genome analyzed and recorded. Church is also involved in doing gene editing in pigs, for the purpose of removing problematic retroviruses which might stand to cause problems in using pig organs as replacement for failing human organs.

Marcy Darnovsky of the Center for Genetics and Society disagrees with the notion that genetic editing is unlikely to result in unforeseen results. "The medical arguments are tenuous and the possible social consequences are grave," said Darnovsky.[25]

In a subsequent article in the Guardian, Darnovsky wrote:

> "The recognition that scientists alone can't decide whether to deploy this society-altering technology is perhaps the summit's most positive outcome. Already, more and more non-scientists are becoming aware of what's at stake for all of us, and realizing that germline gene editing is a social and political matter, not just a scientific one."[26]

John Harris could not disagree more heartily. Harris, a Professor of Bioethics at the University of Manchester, believes that this technology provides the possibility for human enhancement on a grand scale and should be employed as soon as the "wrinkles" are ironed out. Harris has stated, "We all have an inescapable moral duty: to continue with scientific investigation to the point at which we can make a rational choice."

The laws governing gene editing are in many locations inexplicit, to say the least. The UK permits licensed experiments on embryos up to 14 days, but not implantation in a woman. Some British scientists are agitating for a change in these laws. China's laws are considered to be "ambiguous," as are South Africa's, Chile's and Argentina's.[27]

The US government has made it clear it will not fund any gene editing research which involves viable embryos.[28] However, by adopting this policy without passing legislation banning the practice, the US has inadvertently (or otherwise) opened the door for private labs to accommodate rich people who want to have designer babies.

One wouldn't want to state this was the goal, after all. Would one? Designer babies for the wealthy, while the rest of us lump along with our genetic baggage? This begins to sound almost like the engineered societies that science fiction novels warned us about.

The (US) National Academy of Sciences and National Academy of Medicine have issued a press release announcing a "data gathering" meeting in February to study the ethical and social implications of gene editing.

-- December 25, 2015

14

How To Kill a Whole Lot of People: Scripps Scientists Publish How They Made H7N9 Virus More Transmissible

In 2014, a moratorium was placed on federally funded research which involved making flu viruses more lethal. The moratorium was placed after heated debate generated by research published by a Netherlands team, headed up by Ron Fouchier. Fouchier's research had produced a strain of H5N1 which was able to go airborne, thus greatly enhancing its ability to spread. Fouchier focused on the transmission of the disease among ferrets, which are the lab stand-in for people.[29]

Now, scientists in California have published research concerning enabling the human-to-human transmission of the bird flu virus H7N9. This virus strain is of concern to scientists as it has already infected 1500 people and killed 40% of them. H7N9 has not been known, however, to spread easily from human contact.

The article explaining the three genetic changes which need to be made to transform H7N9 into a virtual pandemic agent was published on June 15, 2017 in the journal PLOS Pathogens.[30]

According to Scripps biologist Jim Paulsen, as quoted in an NPR article, "As scientists we're interested in how the virus works…. We're trying to just understand the virus so that we can be prepared."[31]

The NPR article quotes Paulsen as stating he wants next to test the mutated strain on ferrets.

Reuters reported on a number of scientists who were enthusiastic about the Scripps findings. Reuters quoted immunology expert Fiona Culley, who stated that "This study will help us to monitor the risk posed by bird flu in a more informed way, and increasing our knowledge of which changes in bird flu viruses could be potentially dangerous will be very useful in surveillance."[32]

Reuters also quoted virologist Wendy Barclay. "These studies keep H7N9 virus high on the list of viruses we should be concerned about," she said. "The more people infected, the higher the chance that the lethal combination of mutations could occur."

Not all the scientists interviewed were happy about the research. When posed with the question of scientists making the genetic changes in the actual H7N9 virus, David Relman, a Stanford professor of microbiology and immunology, was quoted by NPR as stating, "I would be very hesitant, were they to want to do that. In fact, I would be reluctant to have them do that."

WHAT ARE THE CHANCES THAT THIS RESEARCH MAY BE USED FOR NEFARIOUS PURPOSES?

Since 2001, the US government has poured over $100* billion dollars into what was initially called "Biodefense" but has euphemistically been renamed "Health Security." Many of these programs are dual-use; that is to say the research can be used for either protection or weaponization. Scientists argue that it is necessary to first create the weapon (in this case a pandemic agent) in order to research the cure.

However, the US's record of straightforwardness surrounding her "Biodefense" or "Health Security" programs has been abysmal. The limp-wristed investigation into the anthrax mailings of 2001, in which federal investigators neglected or refused to consider any lab but Fort Detrick as the locus for mailing the anthrax spores — which killed five and sickened over a dozen — resulted in the probable culprit at the Battelle Lab or at US Army's Dugway Proving Ground getting a "Get out of Jail Free" card.

It was less than two years ago when Dugway was caught sending live anthrax through the mail to labs, worldwide. Initially, it was thought that nine labs received the live anthrax. The number soon expanded and it was ultimately admitted that 575 separate shipments of live anthrax had gone out in the span of a decade.[33]

The official excuse, "We didn't know our deactivating equipment wasn't working!" was suspect, given numerous earlier reports that the equipment was faulty.

It has also come to light that the US has been leading the UN around by its virtual nose and providing false information both to the Biological Weapons Convention and also to the 1540 Committee concerning its "Biodefense" programs.

The reality is that the sort of research that delves into how to make H7N9 spread easily and efficiently among humans is the kind of research that should raise substantial alarm.

According to sources in the US government, the moratorium on publishing this type of research is soon to be lifted. Shortly, anyone with two specimen vials to rub together may very well be able to surf the Web and learn how to create a worldwide plague. And in our current technocracy, with its worship of science as an inherent good, there just doesn't seem to be much concern about this.

In 1998, Secretary of State Madeleine Albright said, "Iraq is a long way from [America], but what happens there matters a great deal here. For the risk that the leaders of a rogue state will use nuclear, chemical or biological weapons against us or our allies is the greatest security threat we face. And it is a threat against which we must and will stand firm."

We never found those weapons in Iraq. In our zeal to protect ourselves from bogeymen and "rogue states," we may well have become the very threat that we feared.

--June 18, 2017

*Estimate, official figures not released

15

THE US WANTS YOUR DNA: THE DARK UNDERSIDE OF GENETICS

Recent plans revealed by the Trump administration to collect the DNA of migrants at the border have evoked a significant reaction from the ACLU and other groups. In a recent mass email, the ACLU posited the following as indicative of what could happen if this DNA collection were allowed to progress:

> "The Justice Department is claiming it will help solve crimes, but history shows us that the government often abuses mass surveillance tools to violate fundamental rights."

The ACLU email went on to state:

> "DNA collection could become a normal form of government surveillance – for all of us – if the DOJ moves forward with its plans. Through this new policy, the government will vastly expand its law enforcement DNA database, giving it access to powerful information about the population at large.
>
> "Imagine a world in which the government uses your DNA to determine your likelihood of developing a particular health condition or succumbing to substance abuse, and then conditions your ability to work, have children, travel, or receive benefits on that. Or one in which the government tracks your movement by running the DNA you involuntarily leave behind on every cup, tissue, and more against its database."

Chilling enough. The problem is that the ACLU seems to have forgotten that DNA collection of all Americans is already taking place.

The Newborn Screening Saves Lives Reauthorization Act of 2013—a reauthorization of the 2008 Act—was passed by the Senate by unanimous consent on January 29, 2014.

The Act authorized the establishment of the Advisory Committee On Heritable Disorders in Newborns and Children, and sets up, among other things, a central online clearinghouse for DNA collection data.[34]

A CNN article published in 2010, "The government has your baby's DNA" stated that the practice of state collection of newborn DNA began in the 1960s and is at this point in time universal.[35]

The FBI also maintains a DNA database. The FBI reports that as of September 2019 its database contains over 13 million DNA profiles of convicts, over 3 million of arrestees and nearly a million forensic profiles. (CODIS – NDIS Statistics/Federal Bureau of Investigation).[36]

The ACLU is clearly aware of potential abuses in DNA collection. So apparently, is the Secret Service. According to Ronald Kessler, the author of the 2009 book In the President's Secret Service, a contingent of the Secret Service was assigned to collecting bedsheets, silverware and glasses and other items that President Obama had touched in order to protect his DNA from collection by unfriendlies.[37]

DNA is the fingerprint of life. This unique expression lends itself to not only analysis and cures, as the Newborn Act would suggest, and not only to the resolution of crimes, as the FBI DNA collection efforts would have you believe, but also to weaponization.

In 1970, Military Review published an article entitled "Ethnic Weapons," which discusses genetic differences between ethnic groups as well as known enzyme differences in terms of the prospects of developing weapons of war.[38] Analyzing the relevance of enzyme differences, the article states that:

> "The factual basis of abundant enzyme inhibitors of widely different types can be neglected as little as modern methods for their distribution. They need not be gases in a true sense. Well-studied enzymes represent a small proportion of the total number of catalysts necessary for our vital processes."

In terms of the use of incapacitants in warfare, the article goes on to say that

> "Another prospect may tempt an aggressor who knows he can recruit from a population largely tolerant against an incapacitating agent to which the target population is susceptible. An innate immunity would offer concealment of preparations and obvious advantages in many tactical situations. When the proper chemical agent is used against intermingled friendly and enemy units, casualties may occur in proportions one to 10."

Chillingly, the article concludes as follows:

"Not only the factors have been found, but their inhibitors. Thus, the functions of life lie bare to attack."

This article was published fifty years ago. There have been quantum advances in genetic science since. Concerns are now being voiced that gene weapons (ethnic weapons) are being deployed in Africa and elsewhere. This article, first published in New Eastern Outlook, discusses the indications that the epidemic of hypertension and diabetes in people of color can be traced back to the efforts of the apartheid government of South Africa to create a blacks-only bioweapon.[39]

Other researchers have stated concerns about the weaponization of AIDS and Ebola in terms of their proliferation in Africa.[40]

As stated in a 2002 paper authored by USAF Colonel Michael Ainscough,

"The techniques of genetic engineering began to be developed in the 1970s. In the 1980s, genetic engineering was already a global multi-billion dollar industry."[41]

Ainscough goes on to refer to the following categories as emerging threats:

- Binary biological weapons
- Designer genes
- Gene therapy as a weapon
- Stealth viruses
- Host-swapping diseases
- Designer diseases

The article states that

"The biotechnology exists today for some of these possibilities. Indeed, some genetically engineered agents may have already been produced and stockpiled."

In light of the above, it might behoove us to expand our concerns about migrant DNA collection. Sure, the FBI might just be augmenting its database in case some of the migrants choose to commit crimes while in the US. That is certainly one thing to consider. However, in light of the emerging threat of individual and/or ethnic bioweapons development, and given that the US has already been busted for violating numerous stipulations of the Biological Weapons Convention including weapons development, delivery system development and proliferation, there might be other concerns we need to review.

The stripping of privacy rights since 9/11 has rendered us naked to surveillance and intrusion. The very last frontier of our privacy may, in fact, be our genes. Those who wish to enter the US for economic or political reasons should be aware that what they are giving up in the DNA collection process could very well be the most personal and valuable thing they possess. In fact, Americans have already done so.

--October 25, 2019

16

NORTH KOREA BLASTS U.S.
FOR GERM WARFARE PROGRAM

The government of North Korea has leveled accusations that the U.S. is involved in germ warfare research and intends to deploy bacteriological weapons on a large scale. These accusations came in the wake of the recent revelations that the Pentagon mistakenly sent live anthrax to over 65 labs in the United States and also to labs in Japan, South Korea, Australia, Canada and Great Britain.*

The Korean National News Agency, in a report published on June 4, 2015, called the anthrax "horrible white powder" which has the killing potential of "95 percent." The report stated that "the US secretly introduced anthrax germs into south Korea for its experiment to seriously threaten the existence of mankind..." The report also stated that "The above-said anthrax germ experiments in south Korea are heinous war crimes committed pursuant to the U.S. scenario for world domination."[42]

In a separate release, North Korea called for the responsible American officials to be brought in front of the International Criminal Court.

These statements come on the heels of the recent auction of the Needham Report, published in 1952, which documents the use of biological warfare by the U.S. during the Korean War. This rare copy of the report, officially titled "Report of the International Scientific Commission for the Facts Concerning Bacterial Warfare in Korea and China," was put up for auction by South Korean filmmaker Lim Jong-Tae, who had stumbled upon it several years ago in a British bookstore.

Prior to his purchase, the Needham Report was considered to have been permanently lost.

According to investigative journalist Jeffrey Kaye, who recently put parts of the Needham Report on his website, "The U.S. collaboration with Japanese war criminals of Unit 731 was formally admitted in 1999 by the U.S. government, though the documentation of that has never been published."

---

* The final figure admitted by the DoD was that the anthrax was mailed to 194 labs, worldwide and to labs in all 50 states.

Kaye goes on to discuss efforts to debunk the Needham Report by multiple governments, including the U.S. and the U.K. Kaye writes, "The charges of U.S. use of biological weapons during the Korean War are even more incendiary than the now proven claims that the U.S. amnestied Japanese military doctors and others working on biological weapons who experimented on human subjects, and ultimately killed thousands in operational uses of those weapons against China during the Sino-Japanese portion of World War Two. The amnesty was the price paid for U.S. military and intelligence researchers to get access to the trove of research..."[43]

The Needham Report details U.S. bacteriological warfare in Korea and China. According to the Report, U.S. planes sprayed plague-infected fleas in both China and Korea. Insects and spiders carrying anthrax were also dropped in China. Plague-infected voles were parachuted down by U.S. planes in Korea, and cholera-infected clams were dropped on a Korean hillside apparently in an effort to contaminate a nearby drinking water supply.[44]

Testimonies of captured U.S. airmen were also included as buttressing evidence in the report.

WHY IS ANTHRAX BEING MAILED TO SO MANY LABS, ANYWAY?

The recent reports of the Pentagon accidentally mailing live anthrax to 68 labs in 19 states, as well as to the District of Columbia, Japan, South Korea, Britain, Canada and Australia have resulted in a flurry of attention to the methods used to ensure our collective safety from a potential release. Article after article has appeared in the press in the past couple of weeks discussing the methods by which anthrax is killed and how to ensure that an accidental release does not take place again. One question that is not being asked, however, is why the U.S. government is mailing anthrax to so many labs, worldwide.

According to Inbios, a Seattle lab that was named as a recipient of the live anthrax, that lab did not expect to receive anthrax, live or killed. According to personnel at Inbios, the lab had applied for a potential contract involving detection systems. As part of the winnowing out process, the lab was to receive an unspecified agent at which point it could develop the detection system as part of the bidding process. Inbios states it was unaware that the agent they were being mailed was anthrax.

Stanford University was also named as a recipient of the accidental live anthrax mailing.

According to Lisa Lapin at the Stanford University press office, the Stanford lab is studying immune system response, in order to develop vaccines and treatments for anthrax. Lapin refused to supply a contract number for the Stanford research project, stating only that the contract was with the FDA. A search of contracts with the FDA and Stanford at usaspending.gov did not produce any FDA contracts with Stanford for anthrax research.

According to the CDC, there were 321 "organizations or entities" registered as working with live pathogens, such as anthrax. The Government Accountability Office has stated that within those 321 "entities" are 1495 laboratories, which have been accredited to work with live pathogens, and a much larger number working with inert versions of the same pathogen.

There are at least four events involving accidental release from U.S. labs reported every week.

What Else Is Being Mailed?

According to a recent article published in the Hankyoreh, the U.S. has brought other lethal agents into South Korea without informing its government. The highly dangerous botulinum toxin is also named as an agent brought into South Korea for experiments [45]

Behind all this activity involving agents for germ warfare in South Korea is JUPITR. JUPITR is an acronym for Joint USFK Portal and Integrated Threat Recognition. According to Peter Emanuel, Bioscience Division Chief for the U.S. Army Edgewood Chemical Biological Center, JUPITR was planned as a military project to enable U.S. forces in South Korea to defend against a germ warfare attack from North Korea.

JUPITR involves state of the art biosurveillance, with environmental detectors as well as mobile labs which can quickly determine if a biological threat is at play. According to a 2014 interview with Emanuel, four different agents are being assessed – anthrax, plague, bacillia and botoxin. It was unclear if these four agents were all sent to South Korea for tests.[46]

One of the consistent problems with determining whether or not an offensive germ warfare program exists is the "dual-use" bugaboo. What this means, in a nutshell, is that in order to create countermeasures, whether they be vaccines or detection systems, one must have the germ itself on hand. This could potentially provide a smokescreen for an offensive biological weapons program.

Don't Worry, Be Happy

The U.S. has consistently denied that it was engaged in biological warfare in Korea during the Korean War.

Concerning the allegations involving U.S. germ warfare during the Korean War, Jeffrey Kaye wrote:

> "....the U.S. was not serious about conducting any investigation into such charges, despite what the government said publicly. The reason the U.S. didn't want any investigation was because an "actual investigation" would reveal military operations, "which, if revealed, could do us psychological as well as military damage."

Referencing the recent mailing of live anthrax, Department of Defense spokesperson Col. Warren stated: "We are investigating the inadvertent transfer of live anthrax from a DoD lab from Dugway Proving Ground." A separate DoD statement said "There is no known risk to the general public, and no personnel have shown any signs of possible exposure."[47]

The Department of Defense has reported that at least 31 people have been put on post-exposure treatment.[48]

--July 20, 2015

CREEPING TOWARDS FASCISM

17

HUMAN EXPERIMENTATION RAMPANT IN THE UNITED STATES

I n an article in the New Republic in December, 1998; former UN-SCOM leader Scott Ritter decried Iraq's chemical and biological weapons experiments on human subjects. Wrote Ritter,

> "We had received credible intelligence that 95 political prisoners had been transferred from the Abu Ghraib Prison to a site in western Iraq, where they had been subjected to lethal testing under the supervision of a special unit from the Military Industrial Commission, under Saddam's personal authority."[1]

The stance of the United States and her allies has always been that such experiments bear the watermark of a brutal dictatorship and are never engaged in by the free world.

So when Abu Ghraib again hit the news in 2004, concerning the ongoing torture of prisoners by US forces, the US was swift to act in condemning the reports as constituting isolated incidents and not reflective of US policy.[2]

And then the floodgates opened, with more revelations of torture, CIA "black sites," waterboarding and prisoner rape. And torture became a topic of heated debate.

Those who torture would like you to think that they do not, or that torture is necessary for reasons of "National Security." However, any first year medical student can tell you that torture is unnecessary to gain confessions. All that is needed to obtain such ostensibly highly valued confessions is a good dose of sodium pentothal or another such chemical in the array of truth serum drugs.

What one gains by the use of torture is false confessions. False confessions would be highly valued in the continuing "war on terrorism," to provide proof that acts of terror are being perpetrated by those who are detained.

Abu Ghraib may or may not have been the locus of experiments by the Iraqi leadership. What is certain is that the US is engaged in experiments on its own people, without informed consent, some of which achieve the definition of torture.

The US Continues To Evade the Mandates of Informed Consent

The issue of informed consent was central to the The Doctors Trials at Nuremberg, where twenty German doctors who experimented on Jews and others, often fatally, were tried and sentenced.[3] What emerged from the Trials was the Nuremberg Code, which mandates that experimental subjects be given information about the nature of the experiment and the right to refuse.

The Nuremberg Code, however, remains a recommendation, not a law.

Some of these current experiments run by the United States are taking place within the borders of the US and some are taking place in foreign countries, with pharmaceutical and defense agencies as primary perpetrators.

As an act of apparent damage control following the 1994 disclosures of US radiation experiments during the Cold War, President Bill Clinton produced a memo, lodged in the Federal Register, calling for strengthened protections for human subjects.

These radiation experiments exposed US citizens to high levels of radiation, without informing them of the risks. According to reports, the radiation caused the deaths of a number of the experimental subjects.[4]

Clinton subsequently established an Advisory Committee on Human Radiation Experiments to review reports and recommend ways to prevent further unethical research from taking place in the future.

The Advisory Committee's recommendations included mandating informed consent of all human subjects, among other recommendations. However, the Committee's recommendations were never acted upon. And informed consent, which constitutes the core of the Nuremberg Code, was never codified into law.

Obama Perpetuates the Myth of Legal Protections For Test Subjects

Fast forward to 2010, when another embarrassing experimental project, this time launched by the US Public Health Service in Guatemala, hit the front pages of newspapers. US researchers were reported as deliberately infecting over 1500 human subjects in Guatemala with sexually transmitted diseases. This study took place back in the 1940s and was effectively covered up for over sixty years.

In response to this disclosure, President Obama directed the Presidential Commission for the Study of Bioethical Issues to "determine if Federal regulations and international standards adequately guard the health and well-being of participants in scientific studies supported by the Federal Government."[5]

The Commission reported back in December of 2011 with their conclusions that the current US rules would deter such abuses from taking place again.

The Commission failed to take note that research protocols, classified and otherwise, are lacking an informed consent requirement. What this means is that if, for example, an intelligence agency decides to run an experiment using human subjects, that intelligence agency can waive any necessity to inform the subjects and to gain their consent.

The Commission's report is largely a whitewash. In light of the following facts, it is clear that US nonconsensual human experimentation is rampant. Some of these experiments appear to be classified and some not. In many cases, neither the classified research nor non classified protocols appear to be abiding by the stated need for informed consent.

CHILDREN AS LAB RATS

On January 4, 2002, President Bush signed into law the Best Pharmaceuticals for Children Act, which provides incentives for using children in drug trials. The Act offered pharmaceutical companies a six-month exclusivity term in return for their agreement to conduct pediatric tests on drugs. This Act was quickly followed in 2003 by the Pediatric Research Equity Act (PREA). PREA authorizes FDA to require manufacturers of new drug and biologics products to conduct pediatric studies in certain circumstances.

As a result, drug trials on children have gone through the roof.

An article at medicalkidnap.com states that: "In 2006, they found that there were approximately 45,000 children participating in experiments."[6]

According to Victor Yeung, who is with the Centre for Paediatric Pharmacy Research, The School of Pharmacy, at the University of London, over 50% of medicines used on children are not licensed for use either for the stated disease or for the age group.[7]

As it eventuates, the US government is playing fast and hard with informed consent where children are involved. On the surface, it appears that parents must provide consent for children to be enrolled in drug trials. As it plays out in the real world, however, this is not always the case. Parents are often not given adequate information as to the nature of the drug experiments. And in other cases, when the parents raise questions about their children's medical care, they may find the children taken from them by Department of Children Services.

In some cases, they may even have their parental rights terminated by a court.

In 2013, Justina Pelletier was removed from her parents after an emergency trip to the hospital. Justina, who suffers from a rare mitochondrial disease, was re-diagnosed by a new intern at Boston Hospital with "somatoform disorder," after her parents took her to the Emergency Room with what appeared to be a bad case of the flu. The diagnosis of "somatoform disorder" is a psychiatric diagnosis, which essentially stated that Justina's disease was "all in her head." Her parents were unhappy with Boston Hospital's treatment plan and also with their failure to even consult with her regular doctors and refused to sign off on BH's treatment plan.

At that point, the hospital notified DCF (aka Child Protective Services) and the Pelletiers were effectively blocked from further unsupervised contact with their daughter. Justina was placed in a locked psychiatric unit and Lou Pelletier was charged with contempt of court for speaking about her circumstances to a Boston Globe reporter.

After an extended court battle and after her plight made national news, Justina was finally returned to her parents' care. Concerns that she may have been used in experimental drug trials continue.

The Pelletiers are suing Boston Children's Hospital.

A similar playbook was used against Melissa Diegel, an Arizona mother of two daughters also diagnosed with a rare mitochondrial disease. Diegel has now lost her parental rights after she questioned the treatment plan for her daughters, which was put into place by Phoenix Children's Hospital and Translational Genomics Research Institute.

In court proceedings fraught with secrecy, removal of witnesses from the courtroom, sealed records and attempts to cast Diegel as someone who had "overmedicalized" her two daughters, Judge Kristin Hoffman severed all parental rights of Melissa Diegel and ordered the two girls to be put up for adoption.[8]

As in the case of Justina Pelletier, where her parents were deemed unfit for following the recommendations of the primary physician and not honoring the diagnosis of a new doctor, the Diegel case reveals efforts by Child Protective Services to demonize Melissa Diegel for following one doctor's recommendations for treatment for her two daughters, rather than following the recommendations of another doctor. *

Melissa Diegel states that Hanna and Kayla were enrolled in TGen drug trials.

The willingness of courts to interfere with parental rights when the children in question can be used for drug trials reveals a systemic imperative wherein science will trump the welfare of individual children. At the center of such experimental imperatives lies organizations such as TGen.

Translational Genomics Research Institute (TGen) is situated in a modern, multi-story building in Phoenix, Arizona. It was established in 2002 by Dr. Jeffrey Trent, who served for 10 years as the Scientific Director of the National Human Genome Research Institute (NHGRI) at the National Institutes of Health at the National Institutes of Health (NIH) in Bethesda, Maryland, prior to founding TGen.

TGen's promotional literature states that:

> "TGen is on the cutting edge of translational research where investigators are able to unravel the genetic components of common and complex diseases. Working with collaborators in the scientific and medical communities, TGen believes it can make a substantial contribution to the efficiency and effectiveness of the translational process. TGen's vision is of a world where an understanding of genomic variation can be rapidly translated to the diagnosis and treatment of disease in a manner tailored to individual patients."

However, TGen may also be involved in nonconsensual human experimentation. This reporter has uncovered documentation that the Institute maintains agreements with Phoenix Children's Hospital to refer sick children to the Institute. According to a grant proposal from TGen researcher Dr. Justin Hunter, "Dr. Saunder Bernes, senior pediatric neurologist at Phoenix Children's Hospital (PCH), has agreed to refer Arizona residents with NMD for these studies (see attached letter of support)." The grant was awarded to Dr. Hunter on October 23, 2014.

As at least two sick children, Hanna and Kayla Diegel, were "referred" to TGen with disastrous results for their family unit, one might question whether or not TGen's research programs regularly result in terminating family rights.

Phoenix Children's Hospital has continued to deny any such relationship with TGen, even in light of the documents which have surfaced.

TGen maintains numerous contracts with the federal government, including defense contracts. One of these contracts involves sequencing the genome of Burkholderia pseudomallei, which constitutes a Class B bioterror threat.

71

One of the problems with terminating the parental rights of experimental subjects is that reliable information as to what sorts of experiments are taking place becomes difficult to obtain.

Officials at TGen did not respond to calls from this reporter.

Creating the "Perfect Spy"

Using children as lab rats is not the only human experimentation issue that has reared its head in recent years. Following the Congressional Church Hearings of the 1970s, the US government's program to create the "perfect spy," dubbed MKULTRA, was allegedly disbanded.

However, "mind control" experiments have continued, apparently unabated. After hearing testimony from a number of individuals alleging that they are being electronically harassed with mind-invasive technologies, the President's Bioethics Commission issued a letter stating that it would not investigate such allegations. The letter states that:

> "We would like to clarify for your information that the Commission is not investigating or reviewing any concerns or complaints concerning complaints about ... MKULTRA; COINTELPRO; electromagnetic torture or attacks; organized stalking; remove influencing; microwave harassment; covert harassment and surveillance; human tracking; psychotromic (sic) or psychotropic weapons and radio frequency or military weapons or other claims."

Recent articles at such media sources as businessinsider.com have confirmed the existence of such electromagnetic weaponry.[9] Project Censored, which operates out of Sonoma State University in California, has published a report confirming the existence of neurobiological weapons, directed acoustic weapons, electromagnetic crowd control weapons, pulsed energy projectiles and neural implants, all of which mirror the concerns and testimony of thousands of US citizens who are now alleging that these weapons have been covertly and nonconsensually tested on them.[10]

Justice Is Elusive For Test Subjects

The US continues to hold itself up as the leader of the "free world," even in the face of such abuses of its own citizenry. As the US refuses to honor what one spokesperson called "an 'unaccountable' World Court," chances for those used as test subjects and denied their stated rights to informed consent in experiments to obtain justice remain slim.

A lawsuit launched in 2009 on the behalf of military personnel used as chemical and biological test subjects by the US Army at Edgewood and Ft. Detrick military bases has resulted in a decision by a federal court judge that the Army should keep the subjects informed about "health information relating to their participation in chemical and biological tests spanning five decades." No monetary damages were sought in the lawsuit. In light of the damage to the health of individuals who took part in the experiments – without adequate information as to what the experiments constituted – one might wonder if the best that can be obtained after a seven year court battle is an agreement to share such "health information" with the victims.[11]

While on its surface, Bill Clinton's 1997 memo appears to address the issue of human experimentation, this caveat reveals the opposite:

> "This memorandum is not intended to create any right or benefit, substantive or procedural, enforceable at law by a party against the United States, its agencies, its officers, or any other persons."[12]

Writing for mindjustice.org, attorney Cheryl Welsh states that:

> "...until a federal statute that secures the right of informed consent for anyone subjected to classified human experimentation is passed by the legislature and signed into law by the president, the U.S. government has the power to carry out research projects without his consent and without informing the participants of the dangers or future complications."

Any questions? Sadly, the US government won't be answering them... for the time being, anyway.

--March 27, 2016

* Update: *Melissa Diegel was arrested in 2019 and charged with 8 counts of felony child abuse, alleging that Diegel had her daughters treated for "unnecessary conditions" while in her care. A full five years after the children were removed from her, she was arrested in Florida and faces 144 years in prison. Strangely, the records show that the doctors who treated the children following their removal from their mother continued to treat the girls for the same disorders. No doctors have been charged in this case. Diegel is currently free on $100,000 bail. She has been ordered into yet a sixth psychiatric evaluation by the judge, after five evaluating mental health professionals found her competent.*

18

US: Torture Without Borders

An attorney with the State of California reports being gassed inside her home and taken to a hospital Emergency Room, following repeated incidents of electromagnetic attacks. The attacks take place during an extended court battle over her mother's guardianship.

An anti-police corruption activist in Medford Oregon reports an aerosol attack on her dwelling which causes her to lose consciousness.

An award-winning author pens a memoir concerning how the NSA tried to hack into her mind.

A former intelligence officer lines her apartment with boom boxes in order to drown out chatter of electronic voice weapons. She reports that her mission was successful and the voices have stopped.

Are these women crazy or is the US government now testing its weapons on selected civilians?

Bruised by the Iraq war, the revelations that the US government was involved in torturing detainees hit fast and hard. What were initially some horrific photos leaked from Abu Ghraib soon become a virtual flood of accusations. Prisoners, it appeared, were being tortured by simulated drowning; their genitals electroshocked and the uncooperative were put into tiny spaces and deprived of sensory input.

In his campaign promises of '08, President Obama assured us that torture would cease and that Guantanamo would be closed. However, it is nearly eight years since Obama took office, and the prison at Guantanamo has not closed, nor have renditions to countries agreeable to torture ceased. In 2015, Al Jazeera reported that "More positively for his legacy, the NDAA imposes further restrictions on abusive interrogations and helps fulfill his (President Obama's) original campaign promise to stop torture."[13]

A number of individuals with intelligence backgrounds would disagree. In fact, it appears that, as far as torture goes, some are now asserting that the intelligence agencies are using US citizens for target practice.

ELECTROMAGNETIC WEAPONS

In former intelligence officer Julianne McKinney's seminal 1992 report, entitled "Microwave Harassment and Mind Control," she revealed for the first time a disturbing blip on the intel radar. Citing contacts with people across the US, McKinney details what amounts to covert programs to torture people through use of electronic weapons. And to do so in the targets' (TIs) own homes and wherever they may travel.

McKinney's groundbreaking report cited about 25 individuals who claimed that they were being electronically harassed. It is now twenty-five years later and this number has ballooned to hundreds of thousands, worldwide.

According to Wikipedia, "Electronic harassment, or psychotronic torture, or electromagnetic torture is a conspiracy theory." Wikipedia goes on to determine that "These experiences are hallucinations or the result of delusional disorders or psychosis."

Certainly some of the claims of TIs sound odd ... voices being planted in their heads, being stalked by a multiplicity of strangers and, sometimes, even worse.

However, a review of what is declassified in terms of covert projects reveals a number of operations involving attempts to control or direct human thought, and by consequence therefore to mold behavior. Project Artichoke was one of the subjects of scrutiny in the Church and Pike Committee hearings, which took place in the US Senate and the House of Representatives, respectively, during the seventies. A declassified 1952 memo indicates the aim and scope of Artichoke. The memo states:

> "Can we get control of an individual to the point where he will do our bidding against his will and even against fundamental laws of nature, such as self-preservation?"

The Church and Pike hearings uncovered a multiplicity of "black" projects aimed at accessing the human mind. The surviving records concerning Project Artichoke detail forced drugging, including forced morphine addiction and dosing subjects with LSD, in order to determine vulnerabilities to direction and control under the influence. According to released documents, Artichoke was renamed MKULTRA in 1953.

The US Supreme Court has stated that MKULTRA was concerned with "the research and development of chemical, biological, and radiological materials capable of employment in clandestine operations to control human behavior."

The Church Committee's investigation was hampered by an order from CIA Director Richard Helms to destroy the records relating to MKUL-TRA. As a result of the Church and Pike Committee hearings, MKUL-TRA and related projects were reportedly terminated.

It is the contention of Julianne McKinney – who was an intelligence case officer with the US Army – and scores of others that the projects only went underground, in order to escape further detection and oversight.

Preston Bailey, PhD has noted the following patents for neurological weapons which could produce the sorts of effects claimed by TIs:

THE NEUROPHONE: US Patent # 3,393,279. July 16th, 1968 – a device which converts sound to electrical impulses.

SILENT SUBLIMINAL PRESENTATION SYSTEM: US Patent #5,159,703. October 27th, 1992 — A silent communications system in which nonaural carriers, in the very low or very high audio frequency range or in the adjacent ultrasonic frequency spectrum, are amplitude or frequency modulated with the desired intelligence and propagated acoustically or vibrationally, for inducement into the brain.

HEARING SYSTEM: U.S. patent #4,877,027, 31/10/89 — "Sound is induced in the head of a person by radiating the head with microwaves in the range of 100 megahertz to 10,000 megahertz that are modulated with a particular waveform."

HEARING DEVICE: U.S patent #4,858,612, 22/8/89 — "A method and apparatus for simulation of hearing in mammals by introduction of a plurality of microwaves into the region of the auditory cortex is shown and described."

A further review of the literature uncovers dozens more such patents, including the following:

> A HYPNOTIC INDUCER US3014477 ("The primary object of the present invention resides in the provision of physical means of inducing a state of hypnosis"); AN AUDITORY SUBLIMINAL MESSAGE SYSTEM AND METHOD (US4395600); APPARATUS AND METHOD OF BROADCASTING AUDIBLE SOUND USING ULTRASONIC SOUND AS A CARRIER (US6052336); METHOD OF INDUCING AND MAINTAINING STAGES OF SLEEP IN HUMAN BEINGS (microwaves) (US3884218); and METHOD AND ASSOCIATED APPARATUS FOR REMOTELY DETERMINING INFORMATION AS TO A PERSON'S EMOTIONAL STATE (US3884218).

NONCONSENSUAL CHEMICAL WEAPONS TESTING

Not all the current torture allegations involve electromagnetic weapons, however. The Edgewood Test Vets lawsuit charged that the US Army tested a variety of chemical and biological weapons on soldiers, without gaining their informed consent, from the 1950s on into "at least 1976."

According to the plaintiffs, "In this class action, the Plaintiff class seeks declaratory and injunctive relief only – no monetary damages – and redress for several decades of the U.S. Government's use of them as human test subjects in chemical and biological agent testing experiments, followed by decades of neglect, including:

- the use of troops to test nerve gas, psychochemicals, and hundreds of other toxic chemical or biological substances;

- the failure to satisfy their legal obligations to locate the participants of experiments and to provide them with notice of what they were exposed to and what the possible health effects may be;

- the failure to follow their legal obligations to provide medical care to test subjects for health problems related to the experiments;

- the failure to release the test subjects from oaths of secrecy."[14]

According to multiple claims, such non-consensual experimentation is now regularly carried out on citizens. Some of the individuals claiming "torture without borders" have intelligence backgrounds. Geral Sosbee is a former FBI agent whose career with the agency apparently went sour when he objected to an arrest. He subsequently resigned from the FBI and went on to work as an attorney in El Paso, Texas and as a part-time judge. He also taught at the University level. However, Sosbee states that the Agency's vendetta against him became relentless.

Writes Sosbee:

"…no attention is focused on psychological operations against a targeted person even though a growing number of persons worldwide now testify that they are targeted by ruthless and painful campaigns. No law exists that may stop the type of violent activities in which the FBI and the CIA engage regularly against their Targets, foreign and domestic."

Sosbee has diligently and quite publicly documented his ordeal. In the introduction to his report, Sosbee has detailed an extensive list of methods to torture a target, including not only electromagnetics but also other unconventional weapons. He cites repeated instances of poisonings, some apparently life threatening.[15]

Intelligence agencies have long been known to use poisons against foreign spies. What is of note is that poisons are now apparently being used against domestic US targets.

Sosbee is not alone in his claims of chemical targeting.

Carol Warner is the daughter of former CIA General Counsel, John Warner, who was also pivotal in creating the CIA out of OSS back in the forties. Carol received a Masters Degree in Clinical Social Work from Smith College. She was working as a therapist when a woman walked into her office claiming that she had been groomed by the US government as a "presidential model" sex slave.

This contact launched an avalanche in Warner's life. In a book pending publication, Warner writes: "Sometime after I started training and working more intensively with dissociative identity disorder, I began to be aware I was under intense surveillance." (*Return to the Self*, p. 135)[*]

During the Church Committee hearings in the seventies, her father, John Warner, initially became aware of some of the CIA "black ops" programs involving mind control. In her book, Carol Warner recounts some of the discussions she had with her father at that time and comments on the impact of the destruction of MKULTRA records by Director Richard Helms. She writes:

> "As such, it was abundantly clear to my father and myself back then that the programs would not stop, because Congress never knew about most of them."

Carol Warner's soon-to-be-published book, *Return to the Self*, covers a wide range of issues, including ritual abuse, dreams, spirituality and a discussion of government involvement in mind-altering programs. In disclosing her decision to go public about her own situation, Warner tells us that,

> "I was not going to write about this and the many illegal and unconstitutional activities perpetrated against me since 2008, but circumstances have forced me to revise my decision. Unfortunately, as this near-fatal incident (which I will describe later) dramatically proved to me, there is no safety for me in keeping the knowledge I have gained to myself. I have been told by wise counsel that my only safety is in getting the information out. Unfortunately, it has become radically clear the powers that be do not want the information in this book out." (*Return to the Self*, p. 134)

---

[*]   Carol Warner's book was published in 2017 as *Return: Dreaming and the Psychospiritual Journey*.

She then reveals a number of incidents in Virginia in which her house was illegally entered, one in which her alarm wiring was altered and also where she was followed and stalked. She also describes a number of assaults. An avid outdoorswoman, Warner reveals how she was hiking when she became aware she had been followed into a secluded area. Attempting to elude her stalker, she writes:

> "I kept walking, headed there with my sole focus on finding a good temporary hiding place. Then, out of nowhere, I felt a sting in my right butt cheek. To my utter dismay, I felt myself starting to lose consciousness. Whatever it was that had stung me was powerful and was quickly overtaking me. There was no doubt in my mind that I had been drugged. (CIA development of tranquilizer dart guns became public knowledge with the Church Committee investigation in the 1970s). In a flash I assessed my predicament. Succumbing to the drug was not an option—it would mean certain death."

Warner was able to marshal her strength to survive this incident; however, the efforts against her did not stop. Other stalking incidents reveal that her movements were being monitored, as her stalkers chose to advance against her in various locations with potentially life-threatening results.

Warner also reports the use of chemical agents. She details the following event, while eating out:

> "The soup tasted off, and I didn't eat but a few bites of it. I started feeling horrible immediately, with gastrointestinal symptoms. I felt dizzy and fought to keep consciousness... ...I didn't make it but a few steps. When I came to, I was lying on the restaurant floor, surrounded by paramedics."

The doctor's verdict was chemical — not food — poisoning.

WHY TORTURE PEOPLE AT ALL?

Torture is not a reliable method to gain confessions. Truth serum drugs obviate the necessity for using torture to gain information. In this perspective, the repeated claims by governments that torture is necessary for reasons of intelligence gathering are inadequate to explain torture as an interrogatory tool.

However, torture does desensitize and condition the perpetrator. According to McKinney, somewhere in the ball park of 15-20% of US citizens may be involved — at some level — in using others as target practice. The degradation of society and morality implicit here should not go unnoticed.

In a recent interview, McKinney stated that targets are chosen somewhat at random, although she also believes that these torture techniques are being deployed against specific individuals for retaliation. In her 1992 paper, McKinney stated that,

> "...harassment is beginning to surface as a form of retaliation against persons who try to assist electronic 'harassees.' Retaliation suggests loss of control. Under the circumstances, we are not entirely confident that 'whistleblowers' will continue to be exempted from this type of harassment in the long term."

McKinney now believes that these techniques have resulted in deaths. In response to the question why — why would intelligence agencies use these "torture without borders" technologies on US citizens--McKinney stated that she believes that these are training exercises to prepare the perpetrators for a coming holocaust-level event. Rather than controlling the minds of the subjects, which is a common misconception, McKinney stated that the perpetrators are being desensitized and prepared for participation in a more widespread and devastating scenario.

Her conclusions may be echoed by Carol Warner, who wrote that,

> "If people don't understand the surveillance state is turned on the American citizen, I hope and pray my words will help the reader reconsider. The goal is total full-spectrum control of the populace."
>
> September 5, 2016

19

Going Beyond the Obvious Horror: Lessons From Flint, Michigan

Back in the mid-twentieth century, the city of Flint, Michigan was a bustling industrial town. Home to General Motors car manufacturing plants, Flintonians enjoyed union wages with an average annual income higher than San Franciscans or Chicagoans.[16]

When the General Motors plants began to close in the 1980s, a blue collar work force was left without the blue collar jobs. Unemployment soared. The plant jobs had attracted a largely black population and Flint, once a boom town, became a bust town. In 2011 a state of financial emergency was declared by Governor Rick Snyder. Out of 80,000 industrial jobs, Flint was reportedly left with only 8,000.

Lesson 1: Government disinterested and negligent

It was only after Dr. Mona Hanna-Attisha, an Iraqi immigrant and director of pediatric residency at a local hospital, made public her findings that the children of Flint were being poisoned with lead from drinking water that the government was forced to act. The results of her lead screening documented the profound level of lead in Flint children's systems and made Dr. Attisha an overnight global hero. Said Dr. Attisha in a recent interview, "….when we shared our results at our press conference we were attacked. They were like 'No, this is wrong, you are an unfortunate researcher, you're causing near hysteria, our numbers are not consistent with your numbers.'"

It is due to Dr. Attisha's persistence that the story of the children of Flint being poisoned with lead, an irreversible neurotoxin, was finally brought to light.

One of the disturbing aspects of the Flint situation is how many people at how many levels of government knew about the problem and did not act. Officials at local, state and federal level are implicated in knowing about the leaded water problem and failing to act.

Lesson 2: Flint Is Not An Aberration

As this story gains impetus, reports are coming in from other areas of the country indicating a similar problem with lead in the water. The Chicago Tribune recently ran a story revealing that the aging infrastructure in Chicago is also producing lead-poisoned water.

"More than two years after federal researchers found high levels of lead in homes where water mains had been replaced or new meters installed, city officials still do little to caution Chicagoans about potential health risks posed by work that Mayor Rahm Emanuel is speeding up across the city," reported the Tribune.[17]

An article in The New York Times, published February 8, recites a similar problem with leaded water in Sebring, Ohio. As with Flint, months went by before the city took any action at all. The article cites other such instances in Washington, DC as well as cities in North Carolina, South Carolina and Jackson, Mississippi, where "officials waited six months to disclose the contamination...."[18]

It was reported in January that the Navajo water supply had been poisoned by leakage from uranium mines.[19]

A recent article at philly.com states that "Lead poisoning in PA, NJ, may be worse than Flint." According to the article, government data shows that "18 cities in Pennsylvania and 11 in New Jersey may have an even higher share of children with dangerously elevated levels of lead than does Flint."[20]

The article attributes the Pennsylvania and New Jersey levels to consumption of lead paint chips in older houses.

Lesson 3: Politicians use Flint For Political Currency

Presidential hopeful Hillary Clinton was quick to get on the Flint bandwagon. In an NPR interview, Clinton said, "The idea that you would have a community in the United States of America of nearly 100,000 people who were drinking and bathing in lead-contaminated water infuriates me."

Clinton visited Flint in February and spoke at a local church, calling for Congress to pass an emergency funding bill to help Flint. "What happened in Flint is immoral," she declared. "The children of Flint are just as precious as the children of any other part of America."

However, Hillary's efforts did not achieve the desired result. It was shortly thereafter reported that, as US Senator from New York, Clinton had voted against a bill which would have banned a fuel additive which was contaminating water supplies across the country. MTBE was used to make fuel burn cleaner but was found to be a carcinogen. In 2000, a federal investigation found that wells in at least thirty-one states were at risk for MTBE contamination. The legislation to ban MTBE was passed by Congress in 2005. Clinton voted against the ban.[21]

Apparently, Clinton's campaign promises to Flint fell on jaundiced ears. In the recent primary election in Michigan, Clinton was walloped by presidential hopeful Bernie Sanders. The Republican Presidential candidates have all condemned the failure of government to address the Flint water crisis but have failed to suggest any remedy or assistance.

LESSON 4: CHEMICAL AND BIOLOGICAL ABUSES OF US POPULATIONS ARE EPIDEMIC

The indifference or complicity of various levels of government to the poisoning of Flint, Michigan has historical equivalents. The Tuskegee experiments, in which African American males were put into an experimental study group, without their consent, to track how untreated syphilis affected their health, is a well- known stain on US health policy history.

More recently, a number of prestigious universities were caught using "premies"—babies born prematurely– in experimental studies which ran the risk of causing blindness or death to the infants. The families were not informed of the risks of the studies.[22] Another unplumbed depth of degradation lies in the buried history of A-South, a psychiatric inpatient unit at the posh UCLA medical center in West Los Angeles, California. A-South was a detached unit which was reportedly razed to the ground about ten years ago. It is known that human experimentation was ongoing at A-South, which at least for some period of time only serviced welfare patients.

Officials with the hospital continue to deny that A-South ever existed. It has recently been reported that patients housed on A-South were receiving drugs known to be deleterious to their well-being as well as electroshock therapy in excess of what are considered therapeutic levels. It is also known that A-South patients were refused the right to decline harmful treatment. At least one physician, Dr. Derek Ott, who served as a resident on A-South in the 1990s, has been cited as causing the death of one of his patients.[23]

Ott was reportedly reprimanded by the medical board and did not face loss of his license to practice medicine. UCLA has refused to release names of other physicians who did their residency on A-South.

After the Church hearings in the 1970s, MKULTRA, which was the CIA's experimental program dealing with mind control, was reportedly disbanded. Nicholas West reports in Activist Post that the search for neuro-control technologies has only accelerated.[24]

Lesson 5: What else is in the water?

Lead poisoning lasts a lifetime. Once lead enters the neurosystem, it does not exit. Children exposed to lead face a life sentence of diminished learning capacity, lowered IQ and behavior problems.

Lead contamination is not the only challenge facing US water systems. As of 2006, sixty-nine percent of Americans were serviced by water systems that employ fluoride. Fluoride affects the hippocampus in the brain, inducing docility and passivity in those who ingest it, and was used to dose and daze the denizens of Eastern European concentration camps, during Hitler's reign of terror.

Another item of concern is the use of chloramines to disinfect water. Chloramine is produced when chlorine is added to ammonia. According to Dr. Winn Parker, chloramine is known to cause breast cancer and miscarriages, and can cause further deleterious effects when imbibed by someone who faces health challenges, such as kidney problems.[25]

Recent reports have also raised the bar of alarm on the leakage of pharmaceuticals, such as estrogens, antibiotics and psychiatric medications, into US water supplies.[26] Reports from both the WHO and Harvard University have minimized this as a risk to health. However, articles in medical journals—some going back thirty years—have discussed the problem of antibiotic resistant bacteria in drinking water and the potential effects on public health.

Water is life. As the residents of Flint learned, something as precious as water and human lives can now be subject to politicization, scientific experimental imperatives and even, God forbid, a potential eugenics impetus.

March 21, 2016

20

CANCER, CANCER EVERYWHERE ...
BUT NOT IN THE PRESIDENTIAL SUITE

A recent cancer symposium, with a surgical focus, met in Boston to discuss how surgical oncology is experiencing "an exciting evolution and the ways in which we treat cancer are changing."[27]

However, there are indications that the cure for cancer may have already been found and that those who have it are keeping it close to their chests.

In order to support this contention, which may be seen as alarming and extreme, one must look at the rates of cancer among the general population and compare these to the rates of cancer deaths among world leaders.

And the latter is almost non-existent.

In the US, cancer is the second leading cause of death, exceeded only by heart disease. According to recently breaking news, Australia now lists cancer as its leading cause of death. In the rest of the developed world, cancer is near the top of the list. A recent list published by the World Cancer Research Fund International shows that Denmark leads the pack in terms of cancer rates.[28] Indeed, the list of the fifty countries with the highest cancer rates might lead one to believe that cancer is a disease of prosperity. Conspicuously absent from the list are countries in the Third World—in particular Africa.

Cancer will fell approximately ¼ of all those living in the developed world. However, this particular manifestation of the Grim Reaper gives world leaders a wide berth.

Since 1980, when the exiled Shah of Iran succumbed to lymphatic cancer in Egypt, the deaths by cancer of those leading their nations can be counted on the fingers of one hand. And what is most telling about those on this short list is where they stood on the political spectrum.

Hugo Chavez, the colorful and controversial President of Venezuela between 1999-2013, was a Socialist and prominent adversary of US foreign policy and neo-liberalism. Before succumbing to cancer in 2013, Chavez made a much publicized radio announcement in which he speculated that the US government gave him cancer.

Chavez has been quoted as saying, "Would it be so strange that they've invented the technology to spread cancer and we won't know about it for 50 years?" He is also quoted as saying "Fidel [Castro] always told me, 'Chávez take care. These people have developed technology. You are very careless. Take care what you eat, what they give you to eat … a little needle and they inject you with I don't know what.' "

Since his death Venezuela has crumbled into economic chaos.

Vaclav Havel, who was the last president of Czechoslovakia and the first President of the Czech Republic, is somewhat of a more ambiguous character. While he is seen as being a pivotal player in breaking up the Soviet bloc, and therefore bringing what is popularly termed "democracy" to a formerly Communist country, he may have also been serving US and CIA interests, either unintentionally or otherwise.

In his period of political dissidence, prior to ascending to power, Havel was imprisoned a number of times, the longest incarceration being four years. As President, Havel was instrumental in dismantling the Warsaw Pact and expanding NATO into Eastern European countries. Havel died of lung cancer in 2011 at the age of 75.

Jack Layton, the head of Canada's New Democratic Party, succumbed to "an unspecified, newly diagnosed" cancer in 2011.[29]

The NDP occupies the furthest left of Canada's political spectrum. Indeed, there has never been an NDP head of state in Canada.

So when the NDP swept the national parliamentary elections in 2011, winning 103 seats, the NDP became Canada's Official Opposition. Layton's tenancy as head of the opposition was short lived, however. Layton succumbed to cancer less than four months later, passing on in August of 2011. He had been committed to ousting the conservative Harper government. Following Layton's death, the NDP tumbled from its position and currently occupies third place in Canada's parliament.

As Prime Minister of the tiny island of Barbados, David Thompson could only marginally have been considered a world leader. The population of Barbados is less than 300,000, mostly black. Barbados, also known as "Little England," is an independent state with the British monarch as hereditary head of state.

Thompson was in office from 2008 until October of 2010, when he passed away from pancreatic cancer, one of the most deadly forms of the Big C.

Statistically, since cancer is listed as cause of death in roughly ¼ of all deaths, one might logically expect that one quarter of the US Presidents and one quarter of the US Vice Presidents, to pick one example, would have cancer listed as cause of death. With 44 Presidents and 47 Vice Presidents, one might think that somewhere in the realm of 24 or so might have succumbed to cancer.

However, there are none. Zero. Zilch. A search for cancer as a cause of death for German, French or British leaders in the past forty years produces only one name, that of former French President Francois Mitterrand, who succumbed to prostate cancer in 1996 at the age of 80. Mitterrand was the first French President who was a Socialist and he led the nation for fourteen years, as its longest serving President.

Since the 1972 throat cancer death of Edward VIII—who abdicated the throne in 1936—no members of British royalty have died of cancer.

In October of this year, the World Cancer Leaders' Summit will be convening in Paris, France. The announcement for this Summit states that "The World Cancer Leaders' Summit brings together global decision makers who can shape the way our generation addresses the task of eliminating cancer as a life threatening disease for future generations." Their announcement also states, "The Summit plays a pivotal role in this portfolio of global events by ensuring that the 2020 targets detailed in the World Cancer Declaration are appropriately recognised and addressed at the highest political levels."

However, those at the "highest political levels" are often seen as escaping repercussions for criminal behavior and worse. The idea of the "Teflon-coated" political elite is an idea that has now gained general—albeit grim—acceptance.

Given the probability that the cure may already exist, in light of the unusual lack of incidence of fatal cancers afflicting the powerful, one might want to ask the Summit if the world leaders might be willing to share … please?

--October 31, 2016

21

FORMER FBI ANTHRAX INVESTIGATOR FILES LAWSUIT CLAIMING RETALIATION

Retaliation. It is becoming a rather consistent sub-text in growing numbers of reports concerning US policies—domestic as well as international. On the domestic front, attorneys are being suspended from the practice of law for protesting that the courts are corrupt, an intelligence whistleblower flees the US for safety in Russia and a journalist has been stripped of US citizenship.[30] All these stories have the element of retaliation in common.

And now, we have reports of the FBI retaliating against one of their own former agents, allegedly for criticizing a high profile and troubled investigation. Richard Lambert, former Inspector in Charge of the 2001 anthrax investigation (AMERITHRAX) has filed a lawsuit against former Attorney General Eric Holder, former FBI Chief Robert Mueller and others in the Justice Department, alleging retaliation.

Richard Lambert, whose criticism of the FBI's investigation into the 2001 anthrax attacks became public fare on 60 Minutes, has filed a tort claim in US District Court, alleging that an erroneous legal opinion, written by FBI attorney Patrick Kelly and circulated both within and outside of the FBI, resulted in Lambert's being fired in June of 2013 from the position of Senior Counterintelligence Officer with Oak Ridge National Laboratories, a position Lambert took in 2012 after retiring from the FBI following 24 years of service.

Lambert alleges that Kelly's legal opinion branded him as a criminal for taking a job wherein he had contact with the FBI, without allowing the one year "cooling off" period mandated by law for former FBI employees. Lambert points out in his lawsuit that Kelly misreported the law, which allows former FBI employees to maintain exactly such contact if they are in a position wherein they are "representing the US government." Lambert's position at ORNL– a Department of Energy facility– fulfills this stipulation, he maintains.

Lambert states he reported Kelly's conclusions to the US Attorney's office and to the FBI Office of Professional Responsibility, both of which found Kelly's findings to be "meritless."

In his lawsuit, Lambert maintains that he was singled out for retaliation due to the animus created by his criticisms of the AMERITHRAX investigation, an investigation with which he, as Inspector- in -Charge, was intimately acquainted. He states that in 2006 he provided a "whistleblower report" to the FBI's Deputy Director, with concerns that the investigation was pocked with inadequacies, including understaffing, threats of retaliation should the understaffing be reported to the FBI Headquarters, as well as an extensive cover up of what Lambert calls "daunting exculpatory evidence" concerning the chief suspect, Dr. Bruce Ivins, a Fort Detrick researcher.

Ivins reportedly committed suicide in 2008 before he could be arrested. The FBI has continued to maintain that Ivins was the "anthrax mailer." Letters laden with weaponized anthrax spores were put into the mail in the weeks following the attacks of September 11, 2001, killing five people and sickening at least seventeen others.

Lambert's lawsuit describes some of the actions taken by the FBI and DOJ in efforts to brand him as a criminal in allegedly violating the "cooling off" period. According to Lambert, the DOJ "launched and sensationalized massive criminal probes, which included the dispatch of teams of OIG Special Agents ...who raided and searched Plaintiff's office at Oak Ridge National Laboratory, seized and analyzed Plaintiff's personal documents and effects, and interrogated dozens of Plaintiff's ... coworkers and associates in a wild fishing expedition festooned with prurient inquisitions into the intimate and irrelevant details of Plaintiff's private life and marital status."

The DOJ, however, came up empty handed. No charges were ever filed against Lambert, whose lawsuit claims: "Due to the stigmatizing publicity and notoriety surrounding Defendant (Patrick) Kelly's legal opinion and Defendant's inquisition, Plaintiff has been blackballed with the specter of illegal conduct and ethics violations, unable to gain reemployment despite his submission of more than 70 job applications to various employers."

Lambert is seeking 2.5 million in compensatory damages.

Lambert, who holds a law degree and three Master's degrees, is representing himself. His 24-year career with the FBI included a stint as Assistant Special Agent in Charge at the San Diego Division, Special Agent in Charge at the Knoxville Division and Inspector in Charge of the AMERITHRAX investigation, along with other positions.

Another attorney, Barry Kissin, of Frederick, Maryland, also publicly critical of the FBI AMERITHRAX investigation, was reportedly put on a terrorist watch list.[31] Kissin is in private practice and also writes for the Frederick News Post.   --June 5, 2015

22

DoD's Final Report on Anthrax Fiasco a Whitewash

Rather than examining why live anthrax was mailed to nearly 200 labs, worldwide, the United States Department of Defense "Committee for Comprehensive Review of DoD Laboratory Procedures, Processes, and Protocols Associated with Inactivating Bacillus anthracis Spores" has produced a report which essentially whitewashes the activities going on at Dugway Proving Ground, a military base in Utah.

In Spring of 2015, Dugway was found to have sent multiple lots of live anthrax to a number of labs. As the scandal grew, more and more labs were added to the list of those which received the deadly pathogen, sent via FedEx. The final count of labs receiving the live killer agent included labs in all fifty states and nine foreign countries.

The DoD report, published January 13, states that "A single root cause for shipping viable BA (live anthrax) samples could not be identified. DoD personnel appear to have followed their own protocols correctly." The report goes on to determine that "the committee found inherent deficiencies in protocols for three phases in the production of inactive spores that could lead to non-sterile products: 1) radiation dosing, 2) viability testing, and 3) aseptic operations (contamination prevention)."[32]

The report discusses why post inactivation viability testing did not detect the presence of live anthrax and why spores may have survived the irradiation process. A series of recommendations include "enhancement of quality assurance, a more extensive scientific peer review process, and improvements in program management for inactivation and viability testing of BA." (live anthrax).

Steve Erickson, of the Citizens Education Project in Utah, finds the lack of oversight at Dugway to be problematic. "We've been watchdogging Dugway since 1988," Erickson declared in an interview this past week. He has found the defense base to be "less than transparent," and states that Dugway is "conducting experiments which could be considered to be potentially dangerous and of questionable value."

Erickson remembers that a state committee was formed in the 1990s to oversee Dugway. "It died on the vine," he states. "They simply couldn't get any information out of Dugway as to what they were doing over there."

More Anthrax Fallout At Dugway

And when we say "anthrax fallout," we mean that literally. Dugway Proving Ground has performed open air anthrax experiments going back as far as at least 1955. One of these experiments involved dropping anthrax "bomblets" on live monkeys at the Proving Ground. According to a recent article in the Salt Lake Tribune, the Army failed to document the effectiveness of these tests.[33]

The romance between Dugway and anthrax has been going on at least sixty years. When President Nixon discontinued the US's offensive biological weapons program back in 1969, the only thing that apparently changed was the language of the biological weapons experiments. As it was no longer acceptable to produce weapons grade anthrax as an offensive weapon, the language of the work reported that weapons grade anthrax was produced in order to test countermeasures.

However, with so many national and international labs working on anthrax, it is curious that not even an approved second generation anthrax vaccine has been produced. The initial anthrax vaccine, given to troops in the Gulf War, has been thought to produce "Gulf War Syndrome."

According to a confidential source with former military connections, Dugway Proving Ground has been conducting anthrax experiments in pursuit of weaponizing the deadly germ at least since the 1970s and on through the 1990s, at which point the source no longer had direct access to Dugway. According to the source, some of the biological and chemical agent experiments were taking place in underground structures and some in open air.

Dugway Proving Ground lies on 1300 square miles 85 miles southwest of Salt Lake City in Tooele County, Utah. The sprawling complex, which is dedicated to weapons testing, is actually as large as a small East Coast state.

No One Knows What Is In The Bunkers

There are reportedly entire areas of Dugway which can only be entered in a full protective biohazard or chemsuit. Biological and chemical weapons lie buried in bunkers, deep in the Proving Ground, some of which are simply too "hot" to approach without protective gear. The bunkers, states the source, were originally constructed to store munitions and other weapons and may contain weapons that no one has accurately logged in and therefore are considered too dangerous to dig up.

Recently, Senator Orrin Hatch (R-Utah) sponsored a bill which proposes to withdraw a chunk of land from the Bureau of Land Management and swap it out with other parcels of federal land, in order to "facilitate enhanced weapons testing and pilot training."[34]

Steve Erickson is concerned that this exchange will provide a greater buffer zone for Dugway's tests. "One of the designated parcels, called the Southern Triangle, is contiguous with border of Dugway," states Erickson.

Erickson wants to know why so many labs, worldwide, are working on anthrax. "Making access to these pathogens available to hundreds of labs increases by many orders of magnitude the risk involved," states Erickson. Erickson regrets that the Department of Defense failed to address this issue and calls the DoD report "A missed opportunity at best and a whitewash at worst."

One of the compelling attributes of anthrax is that there is no human to human transmission of the disease. In other words, one may potentially (and safely) infect a target population without risking oneself being exposed to the disease.

--January 27, 2016

23

Book Review:
The 2001 Anthrax Deception

In *The 2001 Anthrax Deception: The Case for a Domestic Conspiracy*, author Graeme MacQueen ties together a considerable breadth of evidence related to both the attacks of September 11, 2001 and to the subsequent anthrax letters, weaving together a tapestry which is compelling and logically coherent.

The anthrax letters, also known as the anthrax attacks or "AMERI-THRAX," were put into the mail in the weeks following 911. The letters, which contained anthrax spores, were sent to both media offices and also to two Democratic U.S. Senators, killing five people and infecting seventeen others.

MacQueen has a Ph.D. in comparative religion from Harvard University and stepped down from his position at McMaster University after over thirty years in order to pursue his activities in justice and peace work. He promotes a thesis that the anthrax letters were perpetuated by a well-coordinated US government conspiracy, implemented by the same parties who were behind the events of September 11. His documentation is compelling in its use of open source material to reveal a pattern and inherent design behind the seemingly chaotic events of that time period.

Writes MacQueen,

> "The documentary evidence relating to the anthrax attacks, when studied critically raises serious questions not only about the FBI's account of the anthrax attacks but also about the U.S. government's account of what happened on September 11, 2001."

MacQueen's logic, in which he not only cogently supports his viewpoint but also shoots down possible alternative explanations for the same events, leads the reader, step by step, through a maze of news reports, disinformation campaigns and perpetrator hypotheses with the studied deliberation of a seasoned detective on the trail of an arch-criminal.

In this case, the arch-criminal would be a group of U.S. government insiders — neo-cons — whose power to exert their collective will on the international and domestic stages has left a trail of tell-tale clues.

The author demonstrates that there was fore-knowledge of the anthrax attacks by a number of Washington insiders, including not only the resident of the Oval Office, President Bush, but also members of the Washington DC press corps. And in the face of such a shocking claim, MacQueen delivers, citing instance after instance, including the 2008 admission by Washington Post columnist Richard Cohen, in which Cohen reveals he was advised to procure Cipro (the antibiotic of choice to combat anthrax) around September 11, before the anthrax letters were even mailed.

There was an initial effort to frame Al Qaeda and Iraq for the anthrax attacks, an effort which soon fell apart under scrutiny. He also cites efforts to tie the alleged 911 hijackers to the anthrax attacks, by their own creation of an ostentatious trail which would implicate them in a subsequent biological weapons attack. Through this and other citations MacQueen advances the thesis that the alleged hijackers were on an intelligence mission to draw attention to themselves prior to the events of September, 2001, in order to provide subsequent "evidence" of their involvement in these later events.

MacQueen also takes on the FBI case against Bruce Ivins, the former Ft. Detrick researcher, whose suicide in 2008 did not terminate the FBI's efforts to criminalize him for the anthrax mailings. Skillfully, MacQueen takes apart the FBI's case against Ivins, revealing it to be weak, unsupportable and duplicitous.

However, the book's claim that the purpose of the anthrax letters was to compel Congress to pass the USA PATRIOT Act does not, to my thinking, provide an adequate explanation for the U.S. government's covert involvement in these attacks. As MacQueen himself admits, both Senators Leahy and Daschle were already standing behind the passage of the PATRIOT Act even before their offices received the spore-laden letters.

The USA PATRIOT Act, passed by Congress and signed into law on October 26, 2001, did indeed change the face of America. The resultant NSA surveillance scandals are, however, only one aspect of the changes wrought by this piece of legislation. MacQueen fails to mention the relevant Section 817 of the USA PATRIOT Act — The Expansion of the Biological Weapons Statute — in which the US changed its existing biological weapons statute *to give itself immunity from violating its own biological weapons laws. The implications of this alteration cannot be emphasized enough.*

And while MacQueen mentions in passing that a U.S. Commission stated that a "serious bioterrorism event" was expected by the end of 2013, MacQueen does not detail the chorus of insiders — including U.S. Senators, members of the Department of Homeland Security, vaccine manufacturers and high ranking officers in the US military — who have also made this exact, disturbing prediction. There is reason to believe that such predictions point to another bioweapons attack, and this evidence of fore-knowledge deserves further scrutiny.

Equally, MacQueen only provides mention that the U.S. has pumped $70 billion into a "biodefense" program in the ten-year period from 2001 to 2011. MacQueen fails to question the nature of this shadowy "biodefense" program, which many commentators now consider to be a covert offensive (weapons) program.

These are concerns which go directly to the question of motive behind the anthrax attacks. If it is true that the U.S. government used the anthrax attacks — indeed, launched the anthrax attacks — in order to ramp up a highly illegal and covert program of biological warfare, then the entire world has been put at grave risk.

Rather than following the "bug" trail, MacQueen chooses to focus on Bush's decision to withdraw from the (nuclear) ABM treaty, announced in December of 2001, thus giving weight to a potential nuclear agenda and threat. By choosing to place his focus here, MacQueen in effect drops the ball right before the goal.

The 2001 Anthrax Deception makes a logically coherent case for a government conspiracy to perpetrate both the anthrax letters and the attacks of September 11. MacQueen has done a masterful job in marshaling the evidence and laying it out in a clear and concise manner. In light of the concerns raised in this review, I would go so far as to say that he got us to third base with this book.

To quote MacQueen, "… *however natural the recoiling of the mind before horrific weapons, this shrinking away from reality must be resisted with 'an act of iron will.'*" For those who would avert their gaze from the knowledge that the U.S. government has attacked and murdered its own citizens in order to further its international and domestic agenda, this book makes an important step towards providing that awareness.

--September 27, 2014

24

Chemical Weapons Allegedly Used Against Political Target in Los Angeles

On more than one occasion of late, the US has hurled accusations against Syrian President Assad for the use of chemical weapons against his own people. Analyses of these gas attacks have raised profound questions about the genesis of the attacks as well as questions as to why the US is so very eager to pin these on Assad—eager enough, apparently, to ignore substantial evidence pointing to other perpetrators.

Now, evidence has come to light that the US may be deploying targeted chemical weapons against her own citizens.

In the wake of the recent report that the US was filing false and misleading reports to the UN 1540 (WMD) Committee, this reporter obtained surveillance videos from a political target in Los Angeles, California.[35] The individual providing the videos is an attorney and was also interned in a US detention camp during WWII as a Japanese American. In the past several years, she incurred a number of legal difficulties during her mother's adult guardianship proceedings. (Her mother was also a former US detainee.) She was falsely arrested (and let go without being charged), fired from her job as an attorney with the State of California and also experienced other legal challenges, such as inexplicable restraining orders. These restraining orders are used regularly against family members who try to protect their loved ones from the ravages of guardianship.

Generally speaking the US has chosen to use the "justice system" to disable individuals, as infamously stated by former Attorney General Eric Holder. As we have seen in some of these legal proceedings, the State has chosen to move very aggressively against some people. Barbara Stone, also an attorney, was the subject of several news articles and was initially arrested for taking her mother out to lunch. Stone is still in an Arizona jail awaiting extradition to Florida.

Another individual who came to the attention of the legal system when he tried to protect a brain injured woman's rights is Pastor Cary Andrew Crittenden, who was again jailed this month in Santa Clara County, California, on contested charges of violating his "OR" release by posting a picture on Facebook of a police officer, now being called a "victim" of Crittenden.[36]

Using chemical weapons against a US target in country, however, is a somewhat advanced form of "extra-legal" abuse. It is not unknown, however. Inventor Stanley Meyer's death by poisoning in 1998 may be one of the more well known such murders.[37] Dozens of other scientists have expired in ways that would raise questions as to whether they also succumbed to chemical assassination weapons.

The surveillance videos provided by the Los Angeles attorney show what appears at first glance to be rain falling on her house. A still from the surveillance videos is provided in the photographs section.

However, a check of all 12 channels reveals that the "rain" does not appear to be falling next door, as revealed on channel 5. In addition, the weather report for Los Angeles for the day in question shows no precipitation recorded.

The attorney, whose name is being withheld from this report, was forced to seek emergency medical care after at least one of these alleged chemical attacks. She set up the surveillance cameras after repeated activity around her home. She has also caught strange light activity. Dr. Katherine Horton, a physicist and directed energy expert, has analyzed these photos and determined them to reveal lasers aimed at the chimney. (See photo section.)

For years, those who reported such weaponry have been called "tin foil hats" in an attempt to minimize and ridicule their reports. These surveillance videos, coupled with the stature and integrity of the individual reporting, might raise alarm.

All told, over 120 video and still files were received from this source.

Former AG Eric Holder, in a letter to Congressman Rand Paul, admitted that there might be some scenarios under which drones could be deployed against US citizens in country.[38] Drones are known to be outfitted, in some cases, with chemical weapons. According to domestic chemical weapons law, military and law enforcement and a multitude of others are exempt from chemical weapons prohibitions, even though the US has signed the Chemical Weapons Convention (CWC) and is tasked with destroying all her stockpiles of these weapons. The inherent conflict between the CWC and Title 18 Section 229 of the US Code, governing domestic chemical weapons activity, has not been attended to or resolved.

Under pressure, Holder later reversed himself.

The LA attorney has reported this attack and others to the FBI and the FAA. There has been no response. If indeed what the LA attorney has caught on her surveillance cameras is a chemical weapons attack, then we have moved another step towards a state of peril.

The chairman of the UN 1540 Committee, Bolivian Ambassador Sacha Sergio Llorentty Solíz, was contacted for comment on the mounting evidence that the US is violating the 1540 Resolution, which governs nuclear, chemical and biological weapons activities.

He has not responded.

--August 16, 2017

BIOWEAPONS:
AT THE BREAKING POINT
OF HISTORY

25

Smallpox: A Deadly Shell Game

The recent announcement by the WHO that it was postponing a decision on destroying the remaining smallpox depositories—one allegedly in Russia at VECTOR and the other in the United States at the CDC—may not have been prompted by what the press has termed a difference of opinion between research groups. In fact, the WHO may have no idea how many labs actually possess the deadly variola virus.

As widely reported, WHO's advisory committee on variola virus research (ACVVR), felt that the stocks should be maintained, as the live virus was still needed to develop antiviral drugs.

On the opposing side, the WHO's advisory group of independent experts to review the smallpox research programme (AGIES) was reported as believing that there was no research justification for holding on to the stocks.

Smallpox has killed over 500 million people in the twentieth century. A sustained global effort at vaccination resulted in the declaration, in 1980, that the world had been ridded of the deadly disease.

However, other considerations besides research protocols may be playing into the reluctance of the WHO to announce the destruction of what it terms the remaining stockpiles of smallpox.

Where are the bugs?

There may, in fact, be far more remaining stockpiles than the WHO has copped to. Case in point is a BSL-3 in Arizona, which has been working on smallpox countermeasures for some time now. In order to create a countermeasure, a lab must have supplies of the disease agent on hand. How is it that the WHO and the CDC "forgot" about the Arizona lab? And how is it that the head of the lab, who was formerly with the CIA, is now denying that his lab possesses the virus, while continuing to tout its work on smallpox countermeasures?

Concerns ramp up when one considers the recent incident, widely reported in the news, where scientists stumbled upon live vials of smallpox, previously unaccounted for, in an unused storeroom in a NIH lab in Bethesda, Maryland. This find effectively negates the WHO's pronouncement on the whereabouts of the remaining samples.

In addition, there were reports in May of this year of the emergence of a smallpox-type disease in the Republic of Georgia, which also raises questions as to the alleged eradication of the disease.[1]

Adding more variables (or variola) to the equation is the fact that, after the breakup of the Soviet Union in the 1990s, many of the USSR's biological weapons scientists ended up out of work and were subsequently lured elsewhere, with promises of high paying jobs in other countries. While some of the scientists, such as Victor Pasechnik and Ken Alibek, defected to the US, others reportedly went to work for various Middle Eastern countries. Conditions under which these scientists were recruited make it likely they were able to bring disease cultures with them to their new employ.

Indeed, following the breakup of the South African apartheid government in the 1990s, concerns were running high that the head of the biological and chemical weapons programme, Dr. Wouter Basson, might well end up peddling his expertise and bugs abroad. Nelson Mandela's new government was so impressed by these concerns that Mandela was persuaded to re-hire Basson, so as to keep tabs on him. Basson had allegedly been involved in the murder of a number of ANC officials, as well as purportedly developing a blacks-only bioweapon. This bizarre arrangement between Mandela and Basson was fairly shortlived, as Basson was subsequently arrested in 1997. Many of the South African BW and CW stockpiles were unaccounted for at the time of the change in government.

WHERE ARE THE LABS?

In a continuing public relations nightmare for the CDC, there were several back-to-back accidents in the same time period as the discovery of the smallpox vials in Maryland. In June of this year, at least 62 CDC employees were reported exposed to live anthrax bacteria after potentially infectious samples were sent to labs which did not have the security protocols in place to handle anthrax.

And then in July, it was reported that the CDC accidentally contaminated a benign flu virus with a highly virulent one. This error resulted in the closure of two CDC-related labs.

In fact, the CDC is even having trouble accounting for the whereabouts of its labs. During a 2011 interview conducted by this reporter with Lori Bane, Associate Director for Policy with the CDC Division of Select Agents and Toxins and Von Roebuck, CDC Public Affairs officer, the two stated that there were only about 250 BSL-3s and six BSL-4s in the United States. In reality, the number of level 3 labs exceeded 1350 at that time and the number of BSL-4s was at least three times the number reported by the CDC.[2]

That the WHO is stalling on issuing a directive to destroy the two reported smallpox repositories may be due to the international body being painfully aware that smallpox is not restricted to the CDC and to VECTOR. It might be accurate to state that the WHO has no idea how many stockpiles remain, and is stalling due to its knowledge that it cannot destroy what it cannot locate. The change in the US's domestic biological weapons legislation in 2001, via Section 817 of the USA PATRIOT Act, may have given the United States leverage to become the biological weapons dealer of the world. If that is the case, then the WHO may be putting its collective head onto a chopping block by announcing the destruction of what it cannot in any likelihood control or even locate.

--July 28, 2014

26

Bioweapons:
At the Breaking Point of History

This November, a meeting will take place in Geneva, Switzerland, in a large hall filled with delegates from around the world. This meeting, which has the potential of affecting every single living person on the planet, will get at most passing mention in newspapers. Some reporters will be present, duly noting which country provided what recommendation and which country approved and which country objected. At the most, this may result in an article on page 18 in the larger, more comprehensive daily newspapers.

The hometown dailies probably won't run anything.

Every five years, the Biological Weapons Convention convenes a Meeting of State Parties at the United Nations in Geneva. Every five years, there is some sort of objection raised by one country or another to the fact that this arms Convention has no mechanism to verify that its member nations are complying with the terms of the treaty and every five years, the US pooh poohs the relevance of concerns about the lack of verification and reporting protocols.

However, this upcoming convening of the BWC in 2016 may be special. For at this juncture, it appears that forces working through the US government, and with knowledge and complicity of other world leaders, are perched on the edge of deploying a biological weapons attack that will simply change the human footprint on the globe.

Despite concerted efforts to keep this from public attention, certain little tells keep popping up. Stories hit the press which should, were we in normal times, result in teams of reporters being dispatched, with all the forensic investigative capabilities that newspapers and magazines used to require of top reporters. As we too well know, the funds for in-depth research have virtually dried up and investigative reporters are now an endangered species.

And in the current political climate, even as disturbing as some of these indicators are, they usually end up being reported as "errors" and any intentionality is buried in the dung heap of denial issued by culpable parties. And in the face of all the other negative news, the real weight of these indicators seems to get lost.

COVERUP OF THE COVERUP

I tem: The US was recently reported as having sent live anthrax to nearly 100 labs, worldwide. The labs receiving the active anthrax were both government and private labs. Did any reporter actually ask why the US is sending anthrax, dead or alive, to so many labs? Did a reporter cull through the spending records available at the government website usaspending.gov to ascertain if any of these labs had unlisted anthrax projects? An unlisted project might well be one funded by the CIA and the implications of a secret anthrax project might well have raised some questions.

What the press did with this story was to dutifully report that the Pentagon stated that the anthrax de-activating equipment at Dugway Proving Grounds, which was the sender to all those labs, worldwide, was examined and fixed.

Does that make you feel better? It shouldn't. Dugway was previously caught about eight years ago sending out live anthrax. No one thought to examine the equipment then?

Item: Speaking of Dugway Proving Grounds, would you sleep any better knowing that Dugway possessed in their labs the very same strain of anthrax that was purportedly used by Fort Detrick researcher Dr. Bruce Ivins, whom the FBI alleges mailed live anthrax to a number of Congressmen and media in September of 2001, resulting in five deaths? Would you sleep better knowing that the FBI refused to investigate personnel at Dugway, instead pinning this crime on the unfortunate Dr. Ivins, who conveniently committed suicide, giving the FBI a "Case Closed" verdict on the mailings? In fact, Ivins did not have the equipment to weaponize anthrax.

Item: Freedom of Information requests concerning biological and chemical weapons are routinely given the deep freeze by the US Military.

An investigative group called Muckrock filed a 2014 FOIA with Dugway Proving Grounds requesting a document named "Cold Death, Chemical Weapons and Means of Mass Destruction." After doing the hot potato with this request between various branches of the military, the agencies simply stopped responding. The FOIA was killed through passive non-compliance with the laws governing transparency.[3]

Similarly, researchers at Muckrock also filed a FOIA for documents relating to "Anthrax File Parke Davis and Co" and received a reply stating the request was denied because it was too broad. The denial was appealed and the subsequent document that was sent to the Muckrock investigator was 100% whited out.

In case you happen to think that the Army really doesn't have certain records or that it is in the best interests of all concerned that these records remain private, consider this:

Item: In 2013, Muckrock filed a FOIA with the Army requesting contracts and copies of reports with mega-contracting firm Booz Allen Hamilton over a certain time period. The reply came back stating that no documents existed. However, a quick visit to the US government contract tracking website, usaspending.gov, reveals 6,766 unclassified contracts with the Army and BAH during the relevant time period, for a total of $4,310,543,269.

Item: This reporter filed a FOIA last year requesting a certain contract between the DTRA, a branch of the US military, and a company called Translational Genomics Research Institute in Phoenix, Arizona. The reply from the FOIA office stated that the DTRA does not recognize or honor the contract numbers listed at usaspending.gov. A second FOIA was then filed using a different contract number. There has been no production of documents to date.

I filed a similar request for a specific contract between the Department of Homeland Security and Translational Genomics. In fact, I filed the request five times. No reply has ever been received.

It appears that access to information is regularly being limited. What we need to understand is why.

Bio=Life

Item: The US government is violating the Biological Weapons Convention and the UN won't do a thing about it.

The violations are multiple and severe. To start with, when the US Congress passed into law the USA Patriot Act, in 2001, a section of the Act made it legal for the US government to violate its own biological weapons laws. In so doing, the US essentially violated the international accord known as the BWC.

The State Department attempted to keep the existence of Section 817 away from BWC oversight. According to State Department official Chris

Park, the US "forgot" to inform the Convention at large about the changes to the US domestic legislation. Any changes in BW legislation must be reported, but then again, as we have seen, there is no mechanism to ensure that states are adhering to their responsibilities under the BWC.

The reactions of UN officials and the Convention at large to notification of the US's violations were reported in a previously cited Activist Post article.[4]

All the way up the UN food chain, the UN Disarmament Affairs officials reacted as if they were being handed an envelope laced with anthrax. And no action was taken.

In the five years since the 2011 BWC convening, we have seen an Ebola crisis, a Zika crisis and continued warnings about emerging threats associated with bird flu and swine flu. If the realities behind Ebola and Zika can be verified, it would appear that testing on civilian populations is well under way. We are becoming conditioned to the emergence of strange and deadly new bugs which have the capacity to kill people en masse. Mainstream news organizations, while assuring as that governments are doing everything in their power to protect us from bioweapons, continue to serve in a dual capacity by reminding as that, as far as pandemics go, The Big One is coming. The double message is clever and contrived: "A major pandemic is looming on the horizon and we did not cause it!"[5]

According to a former employee at Dugway Proving Grounds, who spoke with this reporter under conditions of anonymity, Dugway has been testing biological and chemical weapons for decades. Dugway recently cancelled a media tour which could have reassured us that there is no threat posed by the research ongoing at that facility.

A review of the human rights record of the US indicates that, at this juncture, only certain types of people have rights. This is most clearly in evidence in the lackadaisical response from law enforcement agencies when police kill minorities and in the wholesale judicial disposal of the rights of one of the most vulnerable groups in any society, the elderly and disabled.

If there were to be a globe changing event, from which certain types of people would perish while others remain healthy and intact, a selectively engineered or delivered bioweapon would provide the perfect cover. Both sorts of technologies – race -specific bioweapons and selective delivery systems – now exist.

The signs pointing to future deployments are everywhere now. The only question remaining is will we awaken to history before history ends.

--August 20, 2016

27

Dancing the Apocalypso with the Microbial Gestapo

T he Seventh Review Conference of the Biological Weapons Convention was predicted to be a dud. According to a number of
BWC watchers, the expectations for this conference accomplish-
ing very much at all were quite low.[6]

And if you believe the mainstream media, the only noteworthy event
during the fourteen-day conference, held at Palais Nations in Geneva,
Switzerland, took place on December 7, when Secretary of State Hillary
Clinton addressed the meeting. Clinton's speech highlighted the critical
nature of work being done to protect the world from the spectre of biological weapons, but nixed the idea of launching any verification protocol.[7]
The speech was, according to journalist John Zarocostas, "Pure Bolton."

Echoing John Bolton's speech from a decade prior, Clinton stated,

> "First, we need to bolster international confidence that all coun-
> tries are living up to our obligations under the Convention. It is
> not possible, in our opinion, to create a verification regime that will
> achieve this goal. But we must take other steps. To begin with, we
> should revise the Convention's annual reporting systems to ensure
> that each party is answering the right questions, such as what we
> are each all doing to guard against the misuse of biological materi-
> als. Countries should also take their own measures to demonstrate
> transparency…"

John Bolton was Under Secretary of State for Arms Control and International Security back in 2001 when the US stonewalled the long-awaited
verification protocols, refusing to accept the proposal which was years in
the making.

In a widely quoted speech, Bolton said,

> "Will we be courageous, unflinching, and timely in our actions to
> develop effective tools to deal with the threat as it exists today, or
> will we merely defer to slow moving multilateral mechanisms that

are oblivious to what is happening in the real world…The United States will simply not enter into agreements that allow rogue states or others to develop and deploy biological weapons. We will continue to reject flawed texts like the BWC draft Protocol, recommended to us simply because they are the product of lengthy negotiations or arbitrary deadlines, if such texts are not in the best interests of the United States and many other countries represented here today."

Due to this action, the BWC remains a paper tiger, a treaty in name only, with no means of dealing with violations and no way to verify compliance. 165 nations to date have signed the treaty, which entered into force in 1975.[*]

Yes, if you were to believe mainstream media, nothing happened in the rotunda in Room 18, Building E at the United Nations during those icy days in December. Diplomats from all over the world earnestly debated the merits of proposed language for inclusion in a final declaration,[8] which was agreed upon the last day of the meeting, just before the Convention was scheduled to close. The subjects on the international plate included such items as: Should the declaration "encourage" or "support" universalization? Should smaller countries be expected to contribute any money for the Implementation Support Unit, a superannuated secretarial service for the BWC?

One might be tempted to shake one's head in bewilderment at the best and the brightest laboring over a document which could be seen as fulfilling the poetic prophesy of Macbeth's famous absurdist lament: "Full of sound and fury/signifying nothing." Because, in reality, without a verification and implementation protocol, the BWC is pretty much hot air.

Not all in attendance supported the continued lack of verification. Delegates from India, Iran, Cuba and elsewhere repeatedly and plaintively raised their voices insisting that the Convention get back on track and attend to creating a mechanism to give itself some teeth.

These voices were effectively squelched by the Western "democracies," as the UK, US, Canada, Switzerland and others steered discussion away from verification, advocating instead fiddling around with the unverifiable CBMs. The CBMs ("Confidence Building Measures") are forms on which each country is to self report its research programs, legislation and other aspects of their biological "defense" programs. The utter absurdity of expecting countries to accurately report their own activities on these

---

[*]   As of March 2021, 183 nations have signed the BWC

forms is reflected by the dismal rate of compliance in submissions. Asking the fox to report on his behavior in the henhouse, and calling these unverifiable forms "Confidence Building Measures," is simply not taken seriously by most countries. The low CBM submission rate reflects the level of perceived weight these forms carry.

But was the Seventh Review Conference just a bunch of suits and starched shirts exercising their considerable verbal acuity and diplomatic skills and fiddling around while Rome burns?

The threat of a biological weapons deployment is more severe now than at any other time in recent history. Amidst rumors and allegations of covert bioweapons programs in Iran, Russia, Libya and, of course, the drone of complaints about the "terrorists," the United States has quietly and with studied deception launched a biological weapons program of its own.

The BWC bans the development, production and stockpiling of these weapons of mass destruction, but does not ban research. Currently, there are over 1360 BSL-3's in the US and, while the CDC insists there are only 6 BSL-4's, the actual number appears far higher. The BSLs (biosafety labs) are coded by their containment levels. BSL-4's handle the most dangerous bugs known to man; those for which there is no known cure. The BSL-3's deal with slightly less deadly germs, such as anthrax and plague. According to a report tendered by Edward Hammond, director of the now defunct Sunshine Project, there is no one providing oversight as to the type of research going on in these labs.

Apparently, the Soviet Union had indeed launched an offensive biological weapons program, a fact which came to light in the 1990s, following the dissolution of the Soviet Union. A Soviet scientist who subsequently came over to the US, Dr. Kenneth Alibek, believes that Russia is still involved in developing offensive biological weapons.[9] Questions have also emerged as to whether the research going on at Porton Down in Great Britain may constitute offensive weapons research.

Russia, Great Britain and the US are the depositaries of the Biological Weapons Convention, which is not technically a United Nations treaty agreement, but is rather posited with the Big Three.

This reporter attended the BWC under the mantle of an NGO with the intent of informing the Convention that the United States has violated the treaty and has launched a secret, illegal bioweapons program with intent to deploy. The information provided the delegates, both in a short speech and in subsequent handouts, summarized the following concerns:[10]

1. The United States has amended its biological weapons legislation via Section 817 of the US PATRIOT Act and is now giving its own agents immunity from prosecution for violating the law.

2. The United States has failed to report this change in legislation to the BWC, as it is mandated to do in a politically binding agreement.

3. These weapons are reported to be secretly stockpiled at Sierra Army Depot in Northern California

4. Two separate domestic delivery systems have been delineated— one involving country-wide reconfigurations of water systems, and the other involving impostor pharmaceuticals.

While questions have been raised about some of the general language in 817, the fundamental concern revolves around its final caveat, which states that "c)… the prohibition contained in this section shall not apply to any duly authorized United States governmental activity." A number of attorneys have weighed in on the implications of this peculiar caveat, and some concern has been brewing as to the meaning of this release from culpability.

These concerns were magnified rather than alleviated by the behavior of representatives from the United States during three side events, hosted by Team USA. Dr. Daniel Gerstein of the Department of Homeland Security made a presentation detailing the US's legislative efforts to combat bioterrorism. However, his PowerPoint demonstration featured the older legislation, Title 18 Chapter 10 chapter 175, and did not include mention of the problematic revisions in Section 817.

When this omission was brought to his attention, he mumbled something about needing to check the legislation and quickly moved on to another questioner. When queried about the reports of stockpiles at Sierra Army Depot, Gerstein declared that he didn't believe there was such a military base. It is simple to ascertain that the base indeed exists.

Gerstein made an alarming prediction during his presentation, stating that "we expect a pandemic by the end of 2013." One must wonder how Gerstein could possibly pinpoint a timeline for a pandemic, which is generally seen to be the result of unpredictable microscopic events.

At the second US side event, Selwyn R. Jamison of FBI Bioterrorism responded to a query that the language in 817 constitutes a violation of the BWC stating, "You must be mistaken. The US does not violate treaties." There was no time allowed for a follow-up question, which would have refuted his statement. Waterboarding and the Convention Against Torture come to mind, for starters.

At a third US side event, panel members from Health and Human Services and the Center for Disease Control were asked about plans to triage in event of a pandemic, plans which were first published in Chest, a journal of the American Medical Association, in May of 2008. The triage plans delineate that some people, such as the elderly and those with cognitive disabilities, would of necessity be denied medical care in the event of scarce resources. The Associated Press subsequently picked up on the Chest reports, in a widely published article entitled "Triage plan details whom to let die during a pandemic."[11]

However, both Dr. George Korch of HHS and Dr. Scott Dowell of CDC disavowed knowledge of such triage plans.

While a number of reporters were present for these events, none chose to report on these concerns. Besides some spotty attendance by the mainstream press, the Bioweapons Prevention Project had a reporter present at the BWC, Richard Guthrie. Guthrie produced detailed daily reports as to the events at the Convention; however, he failed to report on the fact that concerns were being raised as to the veracity of the United States' public statements about its compliance.[12] When asked if he would like to be copied on a series of emails between NGO representatives who were pondering the implications of 817, Guthrie replied that there were so many critical issues going on at the Convention that he didn't think it would be worthwhile. He went on to issue an apparent apologia for the PATRIOT Act, saying that he had read it and thought it must have been hastily constructed.

A number of NGO participants took a different view of the relevance of concerns as to the US's compliance, as did a number of state parties, who directly contacted this reporter to express alarm and gratitude for bringing these issues to the fore. Whether or not a state party will act upon these concerns and request the Secretary General to assign an inspection team is as yet undetermined. In the absence of a verification protocol, the only way that an inspection team can be assembled is if a state party contacts the UN Secretary General and requests this.

This reporter also had meetings with several higher-ups at the United Nations. Valère Mantels, Political officer of the Geneva branch of the United Nations Office for Disarmament Affairs, refused to accept documentation from this reporter, saying, "I am not going to burn my fingers turning over documentation to the Secretary General." Peter Kolarov of

Disarmament Affairs declined to meet with this reporter, suggesting the documentation be taken to New York (?). UN Political officer, Bantan Nugroho, also of Disarmament Affairs, did agree to a meeting and was handed a stack of relevant documentation. He declined to take action, cheerfully suggesting that this reporter take Gerstein's 2013 prediction as a personal deadline.

A final meeting with Jarmo Sareva, Director of Disarmament Affairs at the Geneva branch of the United Nations, ended in a stalemate when he informed this reporter, "We are neutral. We do not take sides." When it was suggested that neutrality was a concept useful when there was a debate about facts, but here the documentation amassed may have transcended what could be termed a difference of opinion, he mumbled something about how countries might "use this information for political purposes…." This reporter pushed ahead, stating that "we are not talking about missing money here. We are talking about the possible destruction of human life on a nearly unimaginable scale."

When Sareva did not respond this reporter terminated the meeting.

Early on in the Conference, a member of the US delegation made a comment which may reflect the true nature of the current status of the Biological Weapons Convention. This delegate, Chris Park, an official with the US State Department, reminded the attendees that the BWC itself provides for no meetings after the First Conference. "This Conference has no legal standing," he declared. "We just like each other a lot and so we keep getting together, year after year. But there is no legally binding aspect to anything we do here."

* * *

While in Geneva, I went to see the new Soderbergh film, Contagion. The movie features a scenario in which a pandemic wipes out a big chunk of the world's population. The meta messages in the movie were clear—"Government is good. A pandemic is an accidental natural event and your government is only trying to protect you. Bloggers, however, are evil and opportunistic and not to be believed."

Propaganda, it appears, is not only the dominion of mainstream reporters. Hollywood has gotten into the game, as well, pushing out movies which have a subtext that is frankly poisonous.

So where does this leave us? While no overt movement took place in terms of dealing with the threat posed by the United States, seeds may have been planted. Delegates from a number of countries expressed their concern to me, promising to take the information back to their respective capitals. One can hope that they do.

As I said to Director Jarmo Sareva as I pleaded for intervention, we appear to be cresting on a deliberately engineered attack, under the guise of a circumstantial pandemic, which has the potential of killing untold millions of people. The fact that the delivery systems which have been identified are domestic indicates that the United States is planning to attack selected segments of its own population. Saddam Hussein was hanged for a purported attack on his own people, the infamous gassing of the Kurds. Is the United States now so powerful that no one will attempt to put a stop to this?

Is there a country on earth which has the guts to stand up to America and demand accountability? And while we are waiting to see if a country breaks from the pack, what can we do to protect ourselves?

To be continued...

--January 18, 2012

28

US Lies to UN Concerning Weapons Status

The founders of the United Nations would be heaving convulsively in their graves. A vision, forged out of the carnage of WWII for a world at peace, a world where disputes could be solved by dialogue and diplomacy rather than by bombs, has apparently succumbed to the duplicity of its moving party.

When US President Franklin Roosevelt drafted the initial Declaration of the United Nations in 1941, he penned a document that was a rallying cry for the Allies, in the face of what he termed "savage and brutal forces seeking to subjugate the world." The document boldly stated that "complete victory over their enemies is essential to defend life, liberty, independence and religious freedom, and to preserve human rights and justice in their own lands as well as in other lands…"

In the intervening seventy plus years, the UN has grown in scope and in reach, with divisions and treaty bodies to address trade, commerce, health, communications, human rights, disarmament, food security, refugees, education and more. It now employs over 44,000 people in offices and satellites across the globe.

However, the primary vision of the UN has been subverted by the actions of the leader of the free world. For the US is now actively misleading the UN as to the true nature of her activities.

US Lies About Human Rights

In an earlier article, the attempts by the US to create a false perception to the world human rights community were discussed relevant to specific official statements made by US authorities during the Universal Periodic Review of the Human Rights Record (UPR) of the United States, a cyclical review process held at the UN in Geneva. At the convening of the most recent review in 2015, US officials were found to repeatedly and substantially tweak pivotal statistics and reports in order to cast a false (and benevolent) light upon activities which were uncomfortably redolent of human rights deprivations rather than successes.[13]

Now, we come to assess the truthfulness of the US's reports to the pivotally important UN 1540 Committee. As in reports on her human rights activities, the US has omitted or falsified critical information in her multiple reports to this body.

The 1540 Committee was established as part of the UN Security Council's 1540 Resolution, which attempts to address proliferation of weapons of mass destruction. The 1540 Resolution, which was unanimously adopted on April 28, 2004, calls upon state parties to take several levels of action in order to halt proliferation of chemical, biological, radiological and nuclear weapons. In this article, we will primarily be looking at the US's compliance with non-proliferation of chemical and biological weapons.

BIOLOGICAL WEAPONS LIES

Much has already been written about the efforts by the US State Department to lead the Biological Weapons Convention around by its nose. In 2001, just months before the anthrax attacks of September, the US delegation boycotted the efforts by an ad hoc committee to develop a verification protocol for the BWC. Due to this, the BWC remains with no way to verify compliance by its member parties and no real way to assure that violations can be reported and dealt with.

In other words, the BWC is a whole lot of words, blowin' in the wind.

Rather than any externally verifiable reporting mechanisms, the BWC now relies on "Confidence Building Measures," wherein each state must faithfully self-report to the Convention at large its activities surrounding bioweapons, including any changes in legislation or any stockpiles. As discussed previously, it was confirmed by US Department of State delegate Chris Park in 2011 that the US simply "forgot" to inform the Convention that the Expansion of the Biological Weapons Statute, passed into law as part of the USA PATRIOT Act, gave the US government immunity from violating its own bioweapons laws.

Of equal concern is that the US has actively lied to the BWC. In addition, top UN Disarmament Affairs officials have refused to accept documentation that the US has launched a covert delivery system.[14]

In looking at the US's reports to the 1540 Committee, we find a similar pattern of omissions and outright falsehoods. Nowhere in the US's 1540 National Reports is any mention of the aforementioned legislation, passed in the wake of September 11, giving the US government immunity from violation its own bioweapons laws. Rather, the US's initial 1540 Report, filed in 2004, claims:

> "In accordance with its obligations under several international agreements, the United States has enacted national implementing statutes, which prohibit the illegal possession or transfer of such weapons. In addition,conspiracies, attempts, or threats to use such weapons are also proscribed.[15]

Getting down to the basics of biological weapons prohibitions, the US goes on to assure the UN 1540 Committee that:

> "Under U.S. law, a person may not develop, produce,stockpile, transfer, acquire, retain, or possess any biological agent, toxin, or delivery system for use as a weapon, or knowingly assist a foreign state or organization to do so."

Actually, the US law states that the US government is exempt from these prohibitions.

Since the above cited report was filed in 2004, the US has made no attempts to correct the misperception engendered by these statements. In fact, in the National Report filed in 2013, the US baldly stated that:

> "The United States remains deeply engaged in compliance and assistance activities in support of the Biological and Toxin Weapons Convention (BWC).
>
> Pursuant to terms agreed upon under the Convention, the United States continues to file reports of confidence-building measures with the United Nations Office for Disarmament Affairs." Emphasis added)[16]

As State Department delegate Chris Park admitted, the US has in fact filed incomplete-- and therefore misleading --reports.

Biological Weapons Labs—Leaks Or?

The National Reports filed with the UN 1540 Committee detail some of the other efforts made by the US to advance the mandates of the 1540 Resolution. One of these efforts involves the establishment of labs, worldwide, in concert with the DTRA (Defense Threat Reduction Agency). Over 40 such labs, scattered across the globe, have connections with the DTRA. The National Report states:

"The DTRA Cooperative Biological Engagement Program (CBEP) works with HHS, CDC and the NIH to counter threats of State and non-State actors acquiring biological materials and expertise that could be used to develop or deploy a biological weapon. The programme destroys or secures especially dangerous pathogens at their source and builds partner capacity to sustain a safe, secure disease surveillance system to detect, diagnose and report outbreaks and to work collaboratively with partner country scientists in engagements that support the ethical application of biotechnology to a better understanding of endemic especially dangerous pathogens and their control/prevention."

Not everyone is so sure that these labs are a good idea, or that the labs are even involved in defensive rather than offensive research. And a number of these labs have been at ground zero in recent outbreaks. The recent Ebola outbreak began in the region of the DTRA-connected Sierra Leone lab. A 2015 measles outbreak in Georgia radiated from the area surrounding the Central Reference Lab, a DTRA facility in Tbilisi. A 2016 outbreak of swine flu in Kharkiv, Ukraine, which reportedly killed 20 and sickened hundreds, was uncomfortably close to the location of a lab which had received DTRA project funding.

According to Sputnik News,

"In 2013 in Ukraine alone…. the US created laboratories in Vinnytsia, Ternopil, Uzhhorod, Kiev, Dnepropetrovsk, Simferopol, Kherson, Lviv and Lugansk."[17]

The Russian government has expressed unease about the location of some of these labs. Secretary of Russia's Security Council Nikolai Patrushev has repeatedly pointed out that many of these labs are snuggled up against Russia's borders. In a recent speech to the elite academic institution, Moscow State Institute of International Relations, Russian Foreign Minister Sergei Lavrov's concerns about the US's biological weapons activities were laid out clearly.

As reported in Strategic Culture,

"In his remarks Lavrov said Russia is concerned over the US refusal to negotiate monitoring of biological weapons. According to him, the refusal leads to the conclusion that the US may be involved in biological research for military purposes. This is not the first time Russia expressed its concern over the US covert activities conducted in violation of international law."[18]

Chemical Weapons Lies

The US's official admissions relevant to her compliance with the Chemical Weapons Convention follow a similar path of legalistic omissions. Unlike the BWC, however, the CWC requires that the member states destroy their chemical weapons. According to the mandates of the treaty, which went into force in April of 1997, countries possessing chemical weapons were given a deadline of 2007 to destroy their weapons.[19]

The US did not meet the deadline. An extension was then given until 2012, and again the US had not destroyed her stockpile of CW. Also declaring non-destruction of all stockpiles were Libya and Russia. As now proposed, the US will have until 2023 to accomplish this.

Questions are now being raised as to the nature of the US's domestic chemical weapons legislation and the implications thereof. Akin to the cited concerns about her biological weapons legislation, it appears that the US has given herself a giant sized loophole through which the US or her agents do not need to comply with her own prohibitions against chemical weapons.

Title 18 Section 229—Prohibited Activities—reads thus:

> "(a)Unlawful Conduct.—Except as provided in subsection (b), it shall be unlawful for any person knowingly—
> (1) to develop, produce, otherwise acquire, transfer directly or indirectly, receive, stockpile, retain, own, possess, or use, or threaten to use, any chemical weapon; or
> (2) to assist or induce, in any way, any person to violate paragraph (1), or to attempt or conspire to violate paragraph (1)"

All well and good. However, as we have seen in Section 817 of the USA PATRIOT Act, the devil is usually in the exemptions; that is, who is permitted to violate these laws. And as in the biological weapons prohibitions, we find that the exemptions have left enormous latitude for the US and her agents to violate:

> "(b) Exempted Agencies and Persons.—
> (1) In general.—
> Subsection (a) does not apply to the retention, ownership, possession, transfer, or receipt of a chemical weapon by a department, agency, or other entity of the United States, or by a person described in paragraph (2), pending destruction of the weapon.

> (2)Exempted persons.—A person referred to in paragraph (1) is—
> (A) any person, including a member of the Armed Forces of the
> United States, who is authorized by law or by an appropriate officer
> of the United States to retain, own, possess, transfer, or receive the
> chemical weapon; or (B) in an emergency situation, any otherwise
> nonculpable person if the person is attempting to destroy or seize
> the weapon."

In other words, not only may the US military possess and transfer these weapons of mass destruction, but so can anyone who is attempting to "destroy or seize" the weapon. If this subsection had been written as "destroy AND seize," it might have had a few teeth. But by using the conjunction "OR," the verbiage in this supposedly protective piece of legislation permits ANYONE trying to get their hands on the weapon to do so! As "nonculpable" is not defined in the legislation, this word remains void of meaning.

It should also be noted that law enforcement is also exempt from the prohibitions, as is any other agency of the government.

To sum up, we have no domestic legal protections from these weapons should our government use them against us. In fact, a Syrian chemical weapons victim would have more possibility of redress than one in the US.

In the process of researching this article, this reporter made email contact with the US National Contact for the 1540 Committee, Craig Finkelstein. When no reply was received, I followed up with a phone call. Upon learning that it was I who called him, Mr. Finkelstein immediately disconnected the call. The fact that Mr. Finkelstein is the "Transparency and Media Outreach" Coordinator for the 1540 Committee only ramps up further questions about what the US is up to here.

This article has focused on the BW and CW aspects of US compliance with UN Resolution 1540, which covers CBRN weapons. It is worth noting that, over seventy years since Hiroshima, the world still does not have a nuclear weapons ban. In July of this year, such a ban—the Treaty on the Prohibition of Nuclear Weapons—was passed at the United Nations and will come into effect when signed by at least fifty nations. Of note is that all the nuclear states and all NATO nations (excluding the Netherlands) withheld their vote on the text of the ban.

– August 2, 2017

29

Trump Signs Bill to Further Protect Critical Infrastructure, Including Pandemic Delivery System

President Trump has signed H.R. 3359, the Cybersecurity and Infrastructure Security Agency Act of 2017. The bill is heralded as protecting the nation when in fact this legislation further protects a system which will devastate the nation.

It has been a long standing modus operandi of the United States to disguise its most dangerous projects as protection. Following the events of September 11, 2001 and the subsequent anthrax attacks, the US Congress rushed to pass a massive piece of legislation which ended up putting us in exquisite danger. Embedded in the USA Patriot Act is Section 817, the Expansion of the Biological Weapons Statute, which gave the US government immunity from violating its own biological weapons laws.

The trail begins there. Because what is considered critical infrastructure also entails a bio-chem delivery system, involving a double line water system which has the capacity to selectively deliver toxins to predesignated targets. Blueprints and other documents reproduced in this book lay out the nature of this covert delivery system.

With the passage into law of Section 817, Congress affirmed the right of the US government to deploy biological weapons with immunity.

Now, with Trump signing into law the Cybersecurity and Infrastructure Security Agency Act, we see a similar caveat which again guts our ability to contest this law. According to the CISA law, there is no private right of action.

What this means is that citizens or citizen groups have no right or standing to contest this law.

CISA reorganizes the Department of Homeland Security's National Protection and Programs Directorate (NPPD) into a new agency and prioritizes its mission as the federal lead for cybersecurity and infrastructure protection. It establishes the new agency, Critical Infrastructure and Cyber Security Agency, on the same level as FEMA or the Secret Service.

According to F-Secure advisor Sean Sullivan, "The unanimous passage in the House reflects the seriousness involved – it's beyond partisan politics."[20]

Indeed, the weaponization of critical infrastructure in general and of water systems in particular has been promoted through both Republican and Democrat presidencies. It appears that the project to reconfigure the country's water systems was launched by President Nixon around the same time that Tricky Dick announced that the US was unilaterally abandoning its offensive biological weapons program. Shortly thereafter, the international treaty known as the Biological Weapons Convention (BWC) came into force.

The BWC is largely a paper tiger, without verification or enforcement capabilities. It was under the tutelage of former UN Ambassador John Bolton, now National Security Advisor to President Trump, that the US delegation at the United Nations boycotted the suggested verification protocol, presented to the BWC in May of 2001, just months before the anthrax attacks. Due to this verification boycott, which was affirmed later by Secretary of State Hillary Clinton in her presentation to the BWC in 2011, there is at this juncture no possibility of international intervention with or oversight to any projects by the US government—or any government-- involving potentially dangerous biological weapons activities, including what is clearly a weaponized water delivery system.

The CISA legislation, by removing any right to private action, further circles the wagons and cements the US's ability to covertly deploy through water, which is defined as critical infrastructure, any biological or chemical agent and claim not only immunity but also deny any legal right to protest this through the legal system. Given the covert nature of this delivery system, it is to be expected that the US would claim that the resultant mass deaths to be attributable to a naturally occurring pandemic.

--November 17, 2018

THE PANDEMIC

30

JUSTICE IN THE TIME OF CORONA

"I discovered to my joy, that it is life, not death, that has no limits."
Gabriel Garcia Marquez, Love in the Time of Cholera

One of the casualties of Covid-19 has been our system of justice. The First Amendment to the Constitution, granting freedom of assembly, freedom to practice one's chosen religion, and even freedom of speech is being trampled upon in the face of the corona crisis.[1] The fact that this illness may possibly be no more dangerous than the seasonal flu pandemics of recent years is not apparently part of the official national dialogue.[2]

Michigan recently issued an order for all nonessential workers to stay home, citing the potential to arrest violators on misdemeanor charges. In that state, misdemeanors carry a punishment of up to a year in jail. Other states have issued similar orders, and in Washington DC and elsewhere, you can be jailed and fined for leaving your house. A recent Los Angeles Times article detailed the arrest of a paddle boarder on the coast off of Malibu, among other violators.

Well, we don't want him infecting the fish, right?

In many states, courts are now closed. The DOJ has asked Congress for the suspension of habeas corpus and for the right to detain suspects indefinitely without trial.[3]

Other legal rights are under attack. According to an article in the *Santa Monica Daily Press.*, an effort is afoot in California to waive transparency laws.[4]

> "Noting that city resources and personnel are stretched thin responding to the pandemic, the executive director of the League of California Cities asked (Governor) Newsom last week to "take immediate action to pause certain statutory requirements."

These "statutory requirements" include the public records act and financial disclosures of public officials.

While we are watching our legal protections swirl down the toilet, it is important to remember that they are really pretty illusory. In one recent instance, and in an apparent effort to obscure information relating to a human experimentation project being forcibly inflicted on psychiatric inmates, UCLA Hospitals and Clinics ignored their legal obligations under the California Public Records Act — long before the corona crisis hit.

All was not well in our justice system prior to corona. Fundamentally, our system of justice relies on the integrity of our judges. Long before the corona crisis hit, hard hitting questions were emerging referencing the mounting evidence that state court judges were routinely receiving bribes and pay-offs. It is now appearing that federal judges can be added to the list of those who are similarly self-enriching at the cost of justice.

The revelations that somewhere in the realm of two- thirds of state court probate judges researched had loan histories redolent of money laundering and bribe taking are now being echoed in other "high stakes" courts.

By "high stakes" here we mean courts through which money flows like a virtual waterfall. With 30 trillion dollars set to be transferred from the baby boomers to their heirs, and much of these funds now diverted through adult guardianship courts, these proceedings can certainly be thought of as "high stakes."[5]

(For those not yet aware of the concerns prompted by probate judges' excessive loan activities, a brief Russia Today interview lays out the territory. Airing in 2017, interviewer Sean Stone and I discussed the prevalence of and mechanism by which judges were receiving under the table monies and also the profound reluctance of the law enforcement agencies to do anything about this. Since that interview aired, a number of other journalists have picked up on this story and are also doing the research on judges and their problematic 'loans.')[6]

Tax court could be considered another money-rich venue. A recent investigation of a federal tax court judge, the Honorable Michael B. Thornton, has raised questions as to his loan activity, which appears to be excessive and of concern.

Thornton, who was at one time Chief Tax Court Judge, has been serving as a judge for over twenty years. During this time span, Thornton has encumbered his personal residence with approximately $2.5 million in loans, loans which he pays back very quickly.

For example, the initial mortgage taken out on his property at time of purchase in 1999 was for $428,000 and was paid back in full by 2003. In the meantime, he again mortgaged the property in 2002 for $540,000, a loan which he paid back by 2004. The property was mortgaged twice in

2004—once for $609,000 and again for $592,000. It appears that the loan for $609,000 was satisfied within three years.

This is only a partial rendition of Thornton's loan activity since he ascended to the bench.

As of 2019, Thornton makes $210,900 a year as a tax court judge. Do the math. Given his income and his loan burdens, is Judge Thornton even able to buy himself a hot dog for lunch?

Thornton's wife is also employed, although interestingly enough Judge Thornton has asked the federal Committee on Financial Disclosure to redact her employer's name from his publicly discloseable financial statements, which he is mandated to file each year. We nevertheless located Alexandra Thornton's employer, which is the Center for American Progress, where she is working as Director of Tax Policy.

The Center for American Progress, which publicly details itself as "non-partisan," was founded in 2003 by former Bill Clinton White House Chief of Staff John Podesta, who came again recently to national attention surrounding an email scandal involving leaked emails during his tenure as Hillary Clinton's campaign manager in her bid for the Presidency. Podesta was succeeded as head of CAP by Clinton loyalist Neera Tanden.

In fact, it is well known that the "non partisan" CAP was formed as a left wing think tank to counter the influence of the right wing Heritage Foundation. CAP is funded by The Carnegie Corporation, The Ford Foundation, George Soros, Bank of America, Rockefeller Family and Brothers Fund, Amazon.com and a plethora of other heavyweights.[7]

Thornton's actions on the bench have raised some concerns. In at least one case, Thornton has made decisions on the bench which directly violate due process rights. A petitioner in a case seated in Atlanta filed a motion to dismiss a Notice of Deficiency (NOD) issued by the IRS, alleging lack of jurisdiction. The original case was filed in March of 2018 and the motion to dismiss was filed on August 30, 2019. The response to the motion was filed by the respondent, the IRS Commissioner, on September 10 but never adjudicated by Judge Thornton. Instead, he went forward to trial, ignoring the problematic NOD when in fact the NOD was improperly issued.

The petitioner protested.

In an order dated August 22, 2019, Judge Thornton explicitly issued the following threat to the petitioner:

> "In Harriss vs. Commissioner supra, we warned petitioner that his continuing to advance frivolous or groundless arguments be-

fore this Court could result in substantial penalties in the future. Notwithstanding that warning, petitioner has continued to press the same frivolous and groundless arguments in his motion for summary judgment and in his reply to respondent's response. We strongly warn petitioner again if he continues to press frivolous and groundless arguments before this Court he may expect a penalty pursuant to section 6673 of up to $25,000 for each of these cases."

In other words, if you keep protesting that your procedural rights are being violated you will be fined $50,000.

It has been eight months since the trial and Judge Thornton has yet to rule.*

Thornton was contacted with questions about his loan history and also his failure to adjudicate a pending motion. He has not replied to either set of questions.

The head judge was contacted through the court's media representative with questions about Thornton's loan history and has not responded.

Thornton's loan history, while concerning, is not unique. Using loans as a means to funnel bribes to public officials appears to be very widespread. As justice in the US has been compromised through this and other practices, our mounting concerns about the most recent attack on our justice system through the coronavirus crisis needs to be put in perspective. While it certainly appears that our rights are being taken away, it is more than likely that we did not have the rights in the first place. Not a jolly thought but possibly an important one to remember.

There is a positive side to all this, however. As increasingly people are becoming alarmed at the creeping fascism attached to the official corona virus response, we are seeing that more and more people are asking questions as to what is the motive and intent behind this draconian assault on civil liberties. To paraphrase Paul Anka, "Waking Up is Hard To Do" and we now see people doing so in droves. If we have any possibility of reinstating a free and just society, public knowledge and awareness are absolutely critical.

April 6, 2020

---

* Nineteen months after the hearing on the Notice of Deficiency, Judge Thornton issued a decision in the case discussed herein in March of 2021. While acknowledging that the individual who signed the problematic NOD did not have the delegated authority to do so, Thornton executed some complicated legal gymnastics which both acknowledged this and also granted her a kind of de facto legitimacy. He therefore found for the IRS.

31

A Pandemic Future May Contain a Triangulation of Attacks

There are mounting concerns that the coronavirus has launched a hyperbolic response. The infection mortality rate of the virus is quite low—currently running at .26%, according to one official study.[8] The death toll is also under examination, following the release of information in late August from the CDC that only about 9000 deaths were from coronavirus alone, with co-morbidities contributing to the balance of the deaths.[9] Questions about the integrity of the testing for the virus also persist.[10]

To lock down an entire world, to destroy local economies and devastate the finances of millions, if not billions, of wage earners might be called for under a plague-like scenario, with a death rate much higher than what we are seeing reported. Unfortunately, disputes about the virtues and efficacy of mask-wearing appear to predominate in the discussion. Masks are a symptom but not the disease. They are a symptom of the effort to control and to mandate obedience. For the actual threat, we need to look further.

If the pandemic were to eventuate in a real, honest to God plague-like event, it may very well "ride in" on the purported virus, rather than have any real ties to the virus itself.

There are three potential vectors which hold out this possibility. The first one, which deals with the inherent dangers in vaccines, has been discussed thoroughly in the independent media. Vaccine horror stories indeed abound, from concerns that the adjutants used in vaccines produce neurological damage to reports of vaccine-related deaths in India.[11] Given this history, the fact that the Gates Foundation is so heartily pushing the development of a coronavirus vaccine has many people understandably spooked.

While articles discussing vaccinations as a potential vector for harm now flood the independent media, there are two other portals which, given the pandemic scare at play, also need to be part of the discussion.

One vector is the effect of a quarantine, given the weaponization of the water system.[12] By enforcing a stay at home quarantine on healthy people, one could argue that an attack through the water system could be facilitated — and who would ever know?

The third vector for an attack would be what are called "impostor" or "doppelganger" pharmaceuticals. This has gotten very little press coverage, due very likely to the difficulty in documenting what chemical or chemicals these impostors actually contain. It is known that the intelligence agencies in both the old USSR and in the West maintained a stash of pills that would induce death on consumption by an unwitting target. However, these doubles are now far more widely manufactured and distributed and may account for deaths not only of political targets but also the "dispensables" in nursing homes and other care facilities. Given the nature of a high-profile conservatee's death along with the revelation that the toxicology report was removed from the coroner's file, it is a matter of concern that Charles Castle may have expired from an "impostor."[13]

This reporter has a number of bottles of the "impostors" in her possession and has made strenuous outreaches to laboratories asking for an analysis. To date, no lab has agreed to tackle this.

To center the debate on "to mask" or "not to mask" is, in light of these concerns, a significant diversion. Rather than focusing on the instruments of ensuring obedience and control, the population should consider how best to survive — not only the virus itself, but the three riders coming in on these dark horses. There will likely be no official acknowledgment of any of these riders as potential weapons, as the developing narrative is repetitively geared towards "protection."

To admit that the countermeasures — vaccines, lockdowns and your everyday pharmaceuticals — for this viral pandemic are the actual seat of the danger would be to shatter the narrative at the very juncture when it is entering high gear.

–November 23, 2020

32

WATER AS A WEAPON

In August of 2004, quietly and without fanfare, an article was published on the Los Angeles Independent Media website revealing a plan by the U.S. government to weaponize the water system. The article alleged that this had been accomplished by the construction of a complex system of double lines and mixing capabilities on the main lines. In this manner, certain, pre-selected homes would receive the ordinary water while the targeted homes would receive the mixture. It is the contention of this reporter that the mixture will kill those imbibing the water.

These are shocking, nearly unbelievable allegations. And they hold up under scrutiny.

Nearly three years have passed since the publication of "Public Extermination Project." New information has surfaced supporting these claims. In addition, this reporter has determined some errors in the initial report, which mandate correcting.

A careful reading of Section 817 of the PATRIOT Act, "The Expansion of the Biological Weapons Statute," reveals this to be the umbrella statute which is authorizing this project. While the wording of this statute is somewhat opaque, a diligent scrutiny of the language reveals its true intent. Firstly, this statute is legalizing "delivery systems" and "toxins" under certain circumstances. "Delivery systems" is weapons terminology. "Toxins" are poisons. The statute details when these delivery systems and toxins will and will not be legal.

Poisons, as we all know, are meant to terminate, not enhance, life. There is no mention in 817 of these poisons being utilized as any sort of legally sanctioned punishment for a crime, such as lethal injection. Rather, the statute states that these shall be legal when used for purposes determined as "peaceful, protective, prophylactic or bona fide research."

A dissection of the part of this statute which lists the "restricted persons," who are disallowed from possessing or transporting these delivery systems and toxins indicates that this statute is not authorizing a military operation. The list of restricted persons follows:

"(2) The term `restricted person' means an individual who--

"(A) is under indictment for a crime punishable by imprisonment for a term exceeding 1 year;

"(B) has been convicted in any court of a crime punishable by imprisonment for a term exceeding 1 year;

"(C) is a fugitive from justice;

"(D) is an unlawful user of any controlled substance (as defined in section 102 of the Controlled Substances Act (21 U.S.C. 802));

"(E) is an alien illegally or unlawfully in the United States;

"(F) has been adjudicated as a mental defective or has been committed to any mental institution;

"(G) is an alien (other than an alien lawfully admitted for permanent residence) who is a national of a country as to which the Secretary of State, pursuant to section 6(j) of the Export Administration Act of 1979 (50 U.S.C. App. 2405(j)), section 620A of chapter 1 of part M of the Foreign Assistance Act of 1961 (22 U.S.C. 2371), or section 40(d) of chapter 3 of the Arms Export Control Act (22 U.S.C. 2780(d)), has made a determination (that remains in effect) that such country has repeatedly provided support for acts of international terrorism; or

"(H) has been discharged from the Armed Services of the United States under dishonorable conditions.

Nowhere is there any mention of exclusive military dominion over these delivery systems and toxins. We therefore infer that this is NOT authorizing the use of poisons in warfare against an enemy of the United States of America.

The slam dunk comes a bit later in the text of the law, which states that "the prohibitions contained in this section shall not apply to any duly authorized United States governmental activity."

In other words, the US is given a free pass to violate its own bioweapons law.

So who are the intended recipients of this biological warfare, authorized in this statute? If not an enemy of this country, could it be selected segments of the U.S. population?

We have seen in our country, since 911, the stripping of civil rights that historically accompanies the rise of fascism. Our vote seems to have gone the way of Diebold, and can now be electronically finessed by those who seek to cement their continued governing power. Our privacy rights have been crushed by the "national emergency" that the attacks of 911 established as an ongoing national predicament. Most newspaper editors will acknowledge, at least in private conversation, that they believe their office phone lines to be tapped. Peace groups, and even Quakers, have been under surveillance, and an act as simple and unremarkable as checking a book out of a library now may invoke FBI scrutiny of library records, courtesy of the PATRIOT Act.

The PATRIOT Act had already been written before the attacks of 911, and was waiting in the wings to be trotted out and rammed through Congress. It is not my intention here to attempt an analysis of who the true perpetrators were of the 911 attacks. This has been adequately done by many authors and researchers, including Webster Tarpley and David Ray Griffin. What these redoubtable authors have failed to do is to draw the line of reasoning between the creation of what Tarpley terms "synthetic terror" to the war on Iraq as a position in a global chess game. Rather, the war on Iraq is seen as an invasion for purpose of seizure of oil resources. While it may be that, it is also a whole lot more. And neither Tarpley, Griffin, or any other of the 911 researchers that I am aware of have drawn attention to the implications of 817.

David Ray Griffin has postulated 911 to be a "new Pearl Harbor." Tarpley has compared this event to the Reichstag fires in Hitler's pre-war Germany. While Griffin's analogy to the event that kicked off the U.S. involvement in WWII certainly helps us to understand how governments may either allow or even initiate certain events in order to make war on other countries, it fails in the analysis of what has become, through the PATRIOT Act and the Military Commissions Act, a war on the citizens of the U.S.

Tarpley's comparison between 911 and the Reichstag fires provides a more fertile field for comparison. It is a matter of historical fact that Hitler had his own Brownshirts burn down the German Parliament, then blamed this destructive act on the Communists. This provided a bogus "national emergency" so as to provide a rationale for the stripping of civil liberties necessary for his ascension to dictatorship.

As a result of the false state of emergency, Hitler was granted emergency powers. He ultimately used these enhanced powers to invade Poland, Norway, the Netherlands, France, Belgium as he headed on towards his mission of world control, and to launch an extermination policy within his own country and in the occupied territories. The mass genociding of the Jews, the gypsies, Communists, Jehovah's Witnesses, the disabled, homosexuals and political dissidents has become the modern day standard against which other brutal dictatorships are now measured.

The process of rights- stripping as a result of the creation of "synthetic terror," as well as our imperialistic invasions of the Middle East strongly echo Hitler's prototype. Missing is an awareness of a domestic extermination policy. It is the contention of this reporter that the PATRIOT Act has indeed codified such a policy, via "delivery systems" and "toxins," yet to be deployed. 817 appears to be the slam dunk death clause in the PATRIOT Act.

And if the Jews are, again, one of the primary targets slated for extermination, as this reporter believes, then the destruction of Israel would be a necessary pre-condition for the deployment of the water weapon. Through our invasion of Middle East, we have not only stirred up the cauldron of that region. We have secured multiple bases with proximity to Israel. This could well facilitate the bombing and wholesale destruction of the tiny Jewish state, which our government could then easily blame on Osama bin Laden, Iran, Hezbollah or whatever most convenient fall guy we choose.

The media has gingerly reported the stripping of rights that followed on the heels of the 911 attacks. It is now common knowledge that intelligence agencies can commandeer bookstore records, bug conference rooms and tap phones with impunity. It is NOT common knowledge that the government can, at will and without due process, poison selected U.S. citizens. It is the hope of this reporter that by adequately documenting the plan to use the water system as a weapons system that it may be possible to derail what will otherwise be the worst genocidal attack in the history of the planet.

In order for the water system to be deployed as a selective, finely honed targeting system, it would be necessary for it to be configured in certain ways. First of all, there would need to be at least two water lines in most neighborhoods. One line would provide ordinary water, while the second line would contain the toxins. My research on the water system in such disparate venues as Los Angeles and Spokane has revealed the existence of the double line system.

I have attached two photographs of blueprints from the Spokane water system (Exhibits 1 & 2). These were obtained April 19, 2007, at a public meeting held at Applebee's Restaurant on 29th Street in Spokane. The work in this area has significantly disrupted traffic and access to local businesses. The meetings were held weekly to answer questions of local business owners and residents.

I identified myself as a Sandpoint based writer and requested of Steve Sather, project engineer, a viewing of the blueprints. He immediately complied, and I requested photographing privileges. He assented.

The attached photos, taken that morning, reveal the double line system on 29th Street in Spokane, Washington. This particular project involved the replacement of two water lines—a twelve inch main and a parallel 36 inch main. The onsite foreman, Brian Snipes, who appeared quite uncomfortable with my request to photograph the prints, informed me that the 36 inch line was a transmission line, and not to be tapped. However, the blueprints reveal something pivotal about this system: access line connecting the two lines, every fifty yards or so. According to the specs, both lines were placed 5.5 feet deep. The only reasonable assumption is that the two mains are connected by the access lines.

Snipes had attempted to refute my perception that the two pipes were, in fact, connected. He had informed me that the connective pipe was flexible, and would bend under the second main. The pipe I viewed that day did not, in fact, appear to be flexible.

In 2006, I submitted requests for documents to the Los Angeles Department of Water and Power. Specifically, I requested blueprints from the Ardmore Street Cement Re-lining Project.

The attached letter came back from LADWP, signed by Ronald Deaton, General Manager (Exhibit 3). He stated that certain "sensitive" information would be redacted from the blueprints that would be ponied up to me. Understanding that I would be viewing altered blueprints, I scheduled a meeting in March of 2007. Every print I was given was stamped "REDACTED." However, there were no indications of white-out or black-out on the prints. Aside from a few scattered indications of hydrant valves, there were no other valves detailed on the blueprints. There was also virtually no evidence of service lines from the main(s) to houses or businesses. The infamous second lines were, in almost every blueprint, also missing. In the process of "redacting," it appears that LADWP created entirely new documents for me to view.

I have also attached a recent letter from the City of Santa Monica, in response to California Public Records Act requests for information about the water system (Exhibit 4). Santa Monica was one of the cities initially contacted by this reporter, and the responses to those requests are contained in the link to the original article.

This letter, signed by Eugenia Jimenez for Assistant City Attorney Joseph Lawrence, states that my requests for blueprints and for contracts with private companies are "highly sensitive and jeopardize the security of the City." You may note by re-visiting the "Public Extermination Project" article that Joe Lawrence also put his name to a letter in 2004 stating that there were no records whatsoever on water work in Santa Monica, California. This letter is included as Exhibit 11.

I have also attached two photographs of blueprints of the Los Angeles water system (Exhibits 5 & 6) Through a bit of disingenuous Irish blarney, this reporter was able to view and photograph some of the non-redacted blueprints from the Ardmore Street Project.

I located an ongoing work site, and arrived in the late morning. I had sidled up to a small group of Creamer employees who were digging up a section of the street (both Creamer and Spiniello were awarded sections of the cement re-lining contract). While the crews are buttressing the aging pipes with cement, they are also replacing the manually operated valves with remote controlled valves. This is critical to the deployment of this weapons system. More about these valves a little later on in this report.

I chatted with the forklift operator for a bit. I told him I was a reporter covering infrastructure work. "How boring," he commented. I made a face and agreed. We talked a little, and I asked if I could get a gander at the blueprints. He was agreeable, and asked another crew member to retrieve the plans from the truck. Immediately, I sat down on the curb and began to shoot.

Within a few minutes, he realized that I was photographing the blueprints. He got down off the lift and walked over to me. "Hey," he said uneasily, "I don't know who you are. We are in very strange times. You could be a terrorist....." His voice trailed off.

I smiled at him, as disarmingly as possible, and quickly stuck my cameras in my pocket. "Oh my goodness," I said. "I don't want to worry you. Here, take back the plans." And then I winked at him. "Actually," I said, "I am Osama bin Laden. They shrunk me and gave me a sex change, so the CIA could never find me. Pretty clever, wouldn't you say?"

He laughed. The moment of suspicion had passed. He took the plans back to the truck, and my cameras remained safe inside my jacket pocket.

"Hey, listen to this!" he said to his buddies on the crew. "She's Osama!" Everyone had a good laugh. I stayed a few more minutes, chatting amiably with the guys, then took off, my cameras and photographs secure.

The two attached photos from the Ardmore Street project were taken that day with a cell phone camera and with a standard camera. The second line is in evidence in both photos, which delineate separate streets in the Ardmore Street Cement Re-lining Project.

One of my detractors, a Harry Mobley, of Alton, Illinois, has stated that the existence of two lines is "normal." Mobley writes, ".... but second lines are there already. That's normal. It's a backup to feed around any breaks when certain lines have to be closed down for repair.

This way, the problem affects the least amount of customers."

If that were in fact true, the city would not need to lay down temporary, gutter lines while doing this infrastructure work. As the City of Los Angeles needs to provide a continuity of water service while working on the main lines, and if the second lines were indeed, as Mobley stated, only back-up lines and NOT containing another substance, the temporary gutter lines in evidence in the attached photograph would not be necessary. The city would simply utilize its back-up line, and would not incur the added work and expense of laying down gutter pipe. The attached photograph of a gutter line during a recent cement re-lining project was taken at Washington Boulevard, in Los Angeles, California (Exhibit 7).

The blueprints I photographed in 2006 from the Ardmore Street Project do not appear to be as complete as the ones I first viewed back in 2004, while the City was working on the Washington/La Brea area, nor as complete as the Spokane prints. Engineers, architects and others with access to water blueprints will affirm that there are layers of work that have been done on the underground utilities throughout the years, and different sets of blueprints will reveal varying levels of complexity in delineating the systems. The blueprints I first viewed in Los Angeles, courtesy of an on-site foreman, revealed not only the existence of double lines, but access lines connecting the two lines at regular intervals. This was also revealed in the plans from the Spokane system.

The L.A. plans had also revealed "crosses" in front of every residence on that street. I had incorrectly designated these as "tees" in my first publication on the water weapon. Tees, be they tee fixtures or tee valves, have three ports. Crosses have four ports. The significance of tees and crosses in the water system is that three or more ports provide the possibility to introduce another substance into the primary line.

For purposes of clarification as to the functions of tees, I have attached a photo of an exposed tee, taken at Casa Las Rosas in Los Angeles, in 2005 (Exhibit 8). As you will see, there are three ports, or accesses. As water cannot flow both East/West and West/East at the same time, two of the ports provide for the uninterrupted flow of water in one direction. The third port would allow for the possibility of an introduction of a substance from another line into the main line.

A valve would be necessary to control the introduction of a substance from another source. Without a control valve, the two substances would be freely intermingling.

My original assumption that tee, or three port valves, were involved in this system may not be entirely accurate. Virgil Diaz, who is a sales rep for Mueller, which has acquired U.S. Pipe, advanced my understanding of this system by pointing out that gate valves positioned on tee joints serve the same function as tee, or three port, valves. The same would go for gate valves on cross joints. The red valve depicted in the second photo on the "Public Extermination Project" article is, in fact, a gate valve, which is a two port valve. The first photo depicts a gate valve on a tee joint. These configurations provide the necessary mixing capabilities.

For further clarification, Spirax Sarco provides a quick primer on valves.[14]

The original article had stated that the red valves were manufactured by Tyton. They are, in fact, manufactured by U.S. Pipe. An overview of the officers of U.S. Pipe reveals a very compelling history. Ray Torok, President of U.S. Pipe, previously spent twenty five years at Alcoa, as Vice President and General Manager of the Aerospace Division. Walter Knollenberg, VP of Finance and Treasurer of U.S. Pipe, previously served as Vice President of Finance and Chief Financial Officer of Burns Aerospace Corporation. Aerospace companies are generally known for their government contracts, including spy satellites, etc. It would be an unusual career path from aerospace to plumbing. Unless, of course, there is a direct connection between the satellites and the water system.

And apparently there is. The ROM Communications website provides a diagram which depicts how remote controlled water valves can be accessed off a computer, lap top or even cell phone (Exhibit 9). As shown in the diagram, the originating signal goes into the internet and up to a satellite, which can then relay the signal to the items featured on the left hand side of the diagram. Please note the inclusion of the water valve as a "remote asset" in the far left of the diagram. I have also attached a photo of gate valves stacked up in the City Yard in Santa Monica, California (Exhibit 10). You will note the chalked in numbers on the valves on the bottom row. These appear to be RFID addresses

The ability to control these valves from a remote location is a necessary component of this system. The system has been configured for a mass deployment—therefore, it would be wildly impractical and ludicrously inefficient to attempt to dispatch teams of workers throughout the broad sweep of this country to dig up the streets and manually turn all the valves at the designated time of deployment. The valves would need to be solenoid, or remote controlled. Thus, at the time of deployment, after determination had been made as to which locations house the targets and which will be "passed over," one would need only throw a switch to open the valves. And the American holocaust would be executed, without the victims or the public being any the wiser as to how.

In a taped interview in March of 2006, Ali Sabouni, the Resident Engineer for the Ardmore Street Project, stated emphatically that "There is no such thing as a remote controlled water valve." When further questioned as to how timed sprinkler systems operate, he sputtered, then back-tracked. "Those are small valves," he said, lamely.

Small valves. What a relief. Then we really have nothing to worry about.

For Ali Sabouni, who is in charge of the Ardmore Street Project, one of thousands of such projects across the country, Ali Sabouni, who refused to tell me the country of his birth or where he obtained his Master's Degree in Engineering, Ali Sabouni tells me that remote controlled sprinkler valves are small valves.

I'm sure glad we cleared that up.

--April 21, 2007

33

HOMEWARD BOUND

Driving up to the pumps, I have a distinct experience of entering "No Man's Land." Gas is up over three bucks in Oregon and shows no sign of ever coming down. It strikes me that this feels like an affront, a virtual assault —that the price of gas is actually attacking my ever-diminishing financial reserves, and laying waste that green stuff which constitutes my nest egg.

A confluence of forces are amassing at this point in time, which are keeping folks home much more than in past years. One is the price of gas. Another is the plunge of the dollar, world-wide. My intended trip to Jerusalem and points beyond will be deferred to a later date, for this reason alone.

Other economic realities buttress the decision to stick around home plate. Job insecurity coupled with the spectre of possible home foreclosures ramp up the sense of financial anxiety. The net effect of these conditions is that Americans are more home-bound. Like so many other Americans, I look anxiously to the political horizon to see a sign of change but see only a changing of the guard as our collective economic future marches towards a dark terminus.

At the same time that the economic realities are keeping us close to home, the government is amassing campaigns, in cities across the country, to get us back on tap water and off bottled water.

Why is this of concern?

The proponents of tap cite a number of reasons that they prefer tap to bottled--drinking bottled water contributes to the emission of greenhouse gases (because the water has to be transported); the increasing amount of plastic bottles in landfills; the sapping of aquifers by bottled; and that selling water guts efforts to make safe drinking water a basic human right. There is increasing concern that chemicals leaching from plastic bottles into the contained water may, in fact, be carcinogenic. Numerous reports recently peppered the main stream press alluding to high bacteria levels in bottled water and a low fluoride level in bottled water. Apparently, some people still believe that fluoride is good for you.

The American's Bulletin published an expose back in 2007, citing a cover-up involving a double line water system and the planned use of water as a weapon, authorized under Section 817 of the U.S. Patriot Act. It is the contention of this reporter that 817 is an "umbrella" statute, authorizing a number of poison projects, including, but not limited to, the water weapon.

One of the diabolical aspects of this double line water project is its ability to selectively hone in on its targets. We live in a melting pot, with city council members living next door to rabbis who are living next door to drug dealers who are living next door to political activists.

In order for there to be a "clean sweep," there would need to be a "surgical," incisive attack on the target populations, leaving the non-targets unscathed. The water weapon, with its system of double lines and remote controlled valves, provides the necessary selectivity to accomplish the aims of those dead-set on removing certain elements. Permanently.

And in order for the deployment of this weapon to gain maximum effect, the intended victims should be at home, not gallivanting in France or jet setting across country.

Further information has come to light which substantiates concern that something funky is going on with our water. A couple of years back, a public records request in Medford, Oregon produced a flurry of refusals to turn over information concerning water to this reporter. In a meeting with Medford Water Commission engineer Eric Johnson and public information specialist Laura Hodnett, Johnson refused to turn over the site and utility plans and blueprints for the Lithia Commons, a business development in downtown Medford. Lithia had planned to build their corporate headquarters in downtown Medford, and had done the underground water line work to service this project. Johnson suggested instead that this reporter contact the Lithia Corporation, via Eric Iversen, project manager for Lithia Commons.

Iverson also refused to turn over the records, stating that Lithia, as a private corporation, is not subject to the Oregon Public Records Act. When this reporter, through an extreme effort, did retrieve a portion of the site and utility plans for this project, Iversen sent over one terse message—that he would not communicate any further with this reporter. He referred all questions to Robert Sacks, Lithia's public information specialist.

A nervous Mr. Sacks did get back to this reporter. After quizzing this reporter on her credentials, her newspaper experience, on the type of paper she writes for and why there would be any national interest in the downtown Lithia project, he agreed to answer questions on the plans. He then abruptly reversed himself and refused to honor his agreement.

On July 15, 2008 this reporter met with staff engineer Rodney Grehn and Laura Hodnett, public information officer, both of the Medford Water commission. When I walked out of the meeting, an hour and a half later, I had secured the information I needed to conclusively prove that the city of Medford, through the Medford Water commission, was both supplying altered records to the general public and then denying that these records were redacted or altered.

The meeting focused on the site and utility plans for the downtown Lithia project, detailing the pre-existing water lines in the area between 3rd and sixth streets and between Apple and Bartlett. Under an unfortunately bogus "open and transparent government" policy, the MWC maintains a computer in the front lobby, where a member of the public can copy, free of charge, plats which show where the existing water lines are.

Or some of them, anyway.

The only problem is that the plats do not have complete information, and fail to feature the second line on most, if not all, of the streets.

A careful study of the actual site and utility plans reveals a second line on Third, Fourth and Sixth Streets, running roughly North-South, and Riverside and Bartlett running East –West. Bartlett Street actually showed three water lines, either in the planning or existing phase. The only other East-West running street depicted in these plans is Apple, which contained ambiguous lines.

It was not possible to definitively determine if those lines were water or another utility. In total, seven streets were featured in this plan. One street alone—Fifth Street-- did not ostensibly feature the double line system. The only water conduit apparently in the drawing for Fifth Street was a proposed water line.

Fast forward to the plat, provided by the MWC. The only street on the plat to show the double line system is, in fact, Bartlett.

What does this mean? Why in the world would the city of Medford go to the trouble to pretend to provide information to the public, only to hide evidence of multiple lines under the streets?

I asked Rodney Grehn a direct question at the close of the meeting on July 15. He had already gone over the plans with me, and I had determined which undelineated lines were actually water lines, with Grehn's reluctant assistance. I asked Mr. Grehn, point-blank, if the City of Medford were "redacting" the information offered to the public on the lobby computer.

Rodney Grehn took a deep breath. Almost a minute passed. "No," he said.

Another meeting took place with Eric Johnson and Laura Hodnett. Even when confronted with the information contained in the unaltered plans, Johnson quixotically insisted that the two sets were equivalent. Frustrated by his responses, I asked him if his answers to my questions were governed by the fact that the Critical Infrastructure Information Act, passed in 2002, mandates prison sentences for government employees who reveal information about "critical infrastructure." Of course, water is considered to be critical infrastructure. Or at least the second line is.

At that point, both Johnson and Hodnett suddenly arose and walked out of the room. The meeting was over. And they would not be answering this, or any other question.

This reporter gathered blueprints from several different cities in an effort to substantiate perceptions that the double line system was rampant throughout the United States.

The city of Spokane was contacted for their input on the attached blueprints. These blueprints were photographed at a work site meeting in Spokane, and show with great clarity the double water lines, which are color coded blue.

Initially, I was informed by Spokane that the connective pipe was flexible, which would explain away the perception that the lines look as if they are cross connected. Cross connecting potable with non- potable water is against the law.

When informed that I had been on site and had photographed the connective pipe which was clearly NOT flexible, Marlene Feist of the City of Spokane changed her tune and told me that the two parallel water lines were not at the same depth. This would also mitigate concerns that the lines were cross connected. The only problem here is that the blueprints contained no indication that the pipes were at different depths. In fact, the prints explicitly stated that both lines were placed 5.5 feet deep. Apparently, Marlene wanted me to believe that the blueprints lied.

Other indications point to a cover up concerning water pipes. Larry Chertoff, who is one of the top water guys in the country, was interviewed by this reporter and vehemently denied that the double water line system exists. When emailed the Spokane blueprints attached to this story, he declined further comment.

Larry Chertoff, by the way, is the "secret cousin" of former Department of Homeland Security chief Michael Chertoff. Larry Chertoff is currently a director of Alinda Capital Partners LLC, the largest independent infrastructure private equity fund, and has had more than 30 years experience in the public and private sector working on water projects. He was chief economist for New York City's Environmental Protection Administration. He was also the US correspondent to Global Water Intelligence, as well as an advisor to the NYC Comptroller on watershed protection issues. He is a founding Board member of the Environmental Action Coalition, Water Industry Council and Water Institute of the National Council for Public Private partnering and a member of the National Research Council's Water and Technology Board Committee of Privatization of Water Services in the United States. His son, Ben Chertoff, was an editor at Popular Mechanics at the time that magazine ran its infamous Debunking 911 Conspiracy Theories cover story.[15]

We call Larry a "secret" cousin, for he vigorously denies a familial relationship with DHS Michael Chertoff, although Larry's ex-wife has copped to the fact that they are, indeed, cousins. Michael Chertoff was a co-author of the USA PATRIOT Act, which legalized the governmental deployment of poisons and delivery systems, in the infamous Section 817. Looks like we've got a family affair – Mike makes genocide legal and Larry does the footwork while Ben oversees the propaganda.

Extending the water situation to a global perspective, it is of interest to note that American Water Works, which was up until recently a subsidiary of German blue chip utility corporation, RWE, has been quietly buying up municipal water systems across country. There is water everywhere, and American Water Works wants to own it. AWW currently operates in thirty-two U.S. states, and is considered the largest investor-owned water supply company operating within the United States. AWW now supplies water to 16 million people across America. Apparently motivated by a drive towards acquisition rather than size of the acquired utility, AWW recently bought up the water utility that serves Mountain Top Estates in Middle Smithfield Township, which serves 180 people, and then turned around and acquired SJ services in New Jersey, which serves more than 7200 customers.

RWE maintains a close relationship with Bayer, which was at one point in time IG Farben. IG Farben is known to have manufactured Zyklon-B, used to gas millions of people during the Nazi reign of terror. The chairman of the Board of Bayer, Dr. Manfred Schneider sits on the Board of RWE. The former Executive Vice President of Bayer, Udo Oels, also served as member of the Economic Advisory Board of RWE.

RWE and Bayer are currently partnering on a research project involving carbon dioxide.

IG Farben also supplied the fluoride additives to the water in the concentration camps. Fluoride was known even back then to act on the hippocampus in the brain, rendering those imbibing it passive and docile. In boxing, this is called the old one-two punch, with a modern chemical twist: dull them with fluoride, then move in for the kill...

AWW is not to be confused with AWWA (American Water Works Association), which sets the standards for water systems world wide, including the problematic "double-line" system. The last available public posting of the countries NOT subscribing to the AWWA standards revealed a list of nations generally considered by the Western world to comprise the "axis of evil"--Iraq, Iran, Cuba, the Sudan and Syria. This list was compiled just before the invasion of Iraq in 2002. Having decimated the infrastructure of Iraq with repeated bombings, the U.S. is dutifully rebuilding the water system in that country.

AWWA has launched a campaign to get people back "on tap," that is, away from drinking bottled water and back on the very tap water which may turn deadly, when this project is deployed.

The only questions that remain, as I see it, are these: What is in the second line?

And when is deployment planned?

--February 24, 2011

34

US Water Systems May Be Used for WMD Attack

The National BioWatch Stakeholders' Conference will be taking place this Fall and you can bet your booties that the four day symposium will be an exercise in studied futility.

It is not that the focus of the conference is irrelevant. Hardly that. In fact, the issue of protecting the public from an act of bioterrorism could not be more critical. And it is not that the US government is bumbling around in the dark where private enterprise could step in more efficiently. Even given the recent failure of the Generation 3 BioWatch technology to gain Congressional and DHS approval, the technology at hand for detecting an airborne release is still state of the art.

BioWatch was launched in 2003, prompted by the anthrax laced letters which were put into the mail shortly after September 11, 2001. Letters containing anthrax spores were mailed to several news media offices and two Democratic US Senators, killing five people and infecting 17 others.

BioWatch has been described as "the nation's first early warning network of sensors to detect biological attack."

This is how it works: In about thirty cities across America, filters have been mounted, secret sensors sniffing the air and picking up microbes which will be analyzed on a regular basis at a nearby lab. Should there be a biological weapons release into the atmosphere in any of these cities, alarm bells will ring in the nation's capitol and help will be speeding its way to the afflicted areas.

Critics of BioWatch have pointed to the numerous false positives associated with the program.[16] In addition, other concerns focus on the inability of the sensors to detect underground or indoor releases. Critics have also pointed out that sensors placed in large, polluted cities may fail entirely to detect a biological release.

But on one pivotal issue the critics have remained silent. With billions of dollars reported as having been pumped into BioWatch from its inception, there is little attention being given to the potential for an act of biological terrorism through the nation's water supplies.

The US Water Systems Are Wide Open For A Potential Act Of Bioterrorism

In fact, the configuration of the nation's public water systems, a configuration which contains parallel water mains, would provide the perfect, undetectable delivery system for a bio/chem attack. Blueprints obtained by this reporter—and obtained with some difficulty, it should be mentioned—clearly show two parallel lines running down the street in all cities where blueprints were obtained, cross connected by service lines, which provide water into residences. Remote controlled valves positioned on the second line indicate that whatever that second line contains is being withheld by these valves.

But withheld why, and until when?

The system as it is currently configured would allow for the contents of the second line to dump into some houses while being withheld from others, through the opening and closing of the remote controlled valves. In this manner, whatever is in the second line can be selectively delivered to some residences, while leaving others untouched and uncontaminated.

And those behind this attack could remain safe from its effects. Not so with an airborne release. The automation of this system, provided by the remote controlled valves, would keep the public from being alerted that something was going on with the water system.

It has been suggested that, upon the initiation of a pandemic-level event, quarantines may be imposed. That way, whomever is getting the pathogen pulsed into his residence via the water lines will be assured of getting the maximum dose.

If this sounds like science fiction, consider this: Following the events of September 2001, the US Congress passed a piece of legislation, entitled The Critical Infrastructure Information Act, making it a federal crime punishable by prison time for a government official to reveal information about "protected infrastructure." Given the revelations in this report, this apparently includes information about the second water line. The existence of one water main is all that government officials will generally admit to, even when confronted by blueprints providing evidence to the contrary.

In fact, when the City of Los Angeles was tendered a request for blueprints, they wrote back agreeing to provide redacted blueprints. And redact they did.

The City of Los Angeles provided this reporter entirely new blueprints, constructed at taxpayers' expense, with each and every print stamped

REDACTED. And these prints showed one line and one line only, controverted by blueprints for the same blocks obtained by this reporter through the foreman who was supervising the street work. These other, non-altered prints all showed two parallel water mains.

In other words, the public is not entitled to knowledge about the second line.

National Security Or Keep Them In The Dark?

Given the enormous amount of work that has gone into reconfiguring water systems throughout the US (and apparently the work to reconfigure the system into a double line system began around the time that President Nixon announced that the US was unilaterally abandoning its offensive biological weapons program), the BioWatch program could be viewed as a considerable ... distraction.

Over 40 billion dollars have already been allocated for BioWatch since its inception. How much, do you think, has gone into protecting the nation's water supply?

The Department of Homeland Security has put together a number of BTRAs (Biological Threat Risk Assessments). Not one mention of the risk posed by the double line water system could be found.

The Environmental Protection Agency and Department of Homeland Security assure us of their continued efforts to protect critical infrastructure. According to the 2010 National Infrastructure Protection Plan, Water Sector,

> "...utilities have conducted risk assessments and based on the findings of those assessments, owners and operators have created or updated emergency response plans (ERPs) and implemented numerous protective enhancements.
>
> These enhancements include: (1) improving control of access to utilities; (2) expanding physical barriers against vulnerabilities by installing equipment such as backflow prevention devices in pipes and locks on fire hydrants and manholes; (3) increasing control over access, delivery, and storage of chemicals; and (4) hardening cyber network control systems by installing virus- detection software and firewalls, and in some cases by taking control systems offline."[17]

However, when the EPA was recently contacted with questions about the double-line system and also what sorts of tests were used to ascertain the safety and drinkability of US water, that agency was unable to respond. Robert Daguillard, with the national press office for the EPA, offered a canned and entirely irrelevant reply to direct questions, touting the monitoring systems and various Presidential directives. He declined to respond to the question concerning the purpose of the second line and was also unable to reply to questions related to the type of tests run to ascertain the potability of tap water.

Having been advised that the Spokane blueprint was only one of many, obtained from a number of different cities in different states– all of which delineate that problematic and questionable second line– the EPA spokesperson had only this to say: In an email dated August 7, 2015, Daguillard wrote,

> "The blueprint shows a 36" main and a 12" distribution line with service connections. Based on this generic schematic, EPA cannot provide additional information."

When Pushed To The Wall, "Deny Everything!"

The City of Spokane was contacted and their public affairs officer, Marlene Feist, insisted that the two parallel lines were not connected. The blueprints clearly show that a single service line runs from both pipes—Feist denies this. Other prints obtained at the same photo shoot contain a legend which indicate that both mains are both placed at a depth of 5.5 feet, again supporting the perception that the two lines are connected and that the contents of one or of both can therefore dump into any residence. Feist also refuted the veracity of the written legend on the prints which stated the 5.5 ft depth for both lines, in her continued efforts to deny the reality that the two mains are cross connected and using the same service lines from mains to house.

The FBI maintains a WMD tip line. The individual answering that call declined to speak to a member of the press, instead referring the call to the Press Office.

Ayn Dietrich, the press officer with the FBI area office covering Spokane, stated that she could not release information about the double-line water system.

It appears that an act of biological terrorism or a pandemic-level event, either naturally occurring or engineered, is on the horizon. A number of those-in-the-know, including Microsoft entrepeneur Bill Gates, former Senators Bill Graham and Jim Talent (now with the WMD center in Washington, DC) as well as individuals with the Department of Homeland Security have been tolling the bell, warning of an imminent attack.

Recently, The Guardian newspaper in England also announced the inevitability of a such an event.[18] Predictive programming, such as in the movie Contagion, assure us that the US government is the "good guy" and will do everything in its power to protect us when "The Big One" hits.

One has to ask, though. With all this moolah being funneled into protecting the citizenry from an airborne attack and unknown billions of dollars having been spent to reconfigure water systems to provide a covert delivery system for a waterborne attack, one does have to ask.

And this is the one question which no one in the US government appears able to answer:

Hey buddy, what's that second line for?

--August 24, 2015

35

Is Covid-19 "The Big One" Or Just A "Dry Run?"

Let's face facts. As viruses go, the coronavirus is likely a dud. Its mortality rate is low, though its contagion factor appears to be substantial. Compared to the normal yearly death toll from the flu, Covid-19 appears to be in the same ballpark.[19]

Low Mortality Except For "Useless Eaters"

Those who have succumbed to Covid-19 largely comprise the elderly. And the fact is that the US (and many of her Western cohorts) do not give a hoot about the old. Why else would the US be so intent on passing euthanasia laws as well as instituting such notoriously abusive practices as court-authorized adult guardianships, which are not only devastating to a senior's nest egg but very often fatal to the senior so afflicted?

Numerous physicians and nurses have now come forward detailing the pressures being levied to declare non-Covid deaths as Covid deaths. The pressures include ample grants to hospitals for each diagnosis of Covid as well as $29,000 for each patient placed on a ventilator. In addition, hospitals and doctors are urged, via written guidelines, to designate deaths as due to Covid when they are not.

Several years ago, the CDC, the Department of Homeland Security, Health and Human Services and some heavy weights from prestigious universities put their heads together and issued triage protocols, should an epidemic be declared. The triage plans explicitly advised that in the case of a pandemic and limited medical resources, the old and the sick should be denied medical treatment. Other countries, including euthanasia-happy Canada, have similar triage protocols.

So other than potentially culling some senior citizens from the Book of Life, what are the other effects of the coronavirus hysteria?

Why A "Test Run"?

Apparently, this coronavirus is not "The Big One." However, the response by governments and the UN is of such a tenor that one might think it is. And in fact, it may indeed morph into something far worse than what we have seen.

And it may provide a staging platform for "The Big One."

The coronavirus does provide an opportunity to test and/or refine policies and real-time effects of a contagion. These policies include quarantines, closed borders and further intrusions and violations of citizens' privacy rights. The effects could allow ample data for studies of citizen compliance and market research.

We Have No Legal Protection From A State-Sponsored Bioweapons Attack

There are no real national or international legal mechanisms that would protect us from such a bioweapons test, or that would curtail the US from launching The Big One. The toothless, dysfunctional international accord known as the Biological Weapons Convention was launched in 1975 and to this day has no enforcement or verification protocol. As discussed previously, we can thank the US delegation to the Convention, led by John Bolton, for that.

Fast forward to the anthrax attacks of 2001, handily attributed to a Fort Detrick scientist who conveniently committed suicide before he could be charged. As a result of the anthrax attacks, the US government has poured billions of dollars annually into a shadowy and unaccountable biological weapons program. The only publicly available numbers relate to "citizen biodefense"--roughly $6-7 billion a year. No figures revealing DoD, DHS or other military endowments are available.

Dr. Daniel Gerstein (remember him from the 2011 BWC—the DHS Sierra Army Depot denier?) recently agreed to discuss the funding for "biodefense." After explaining that the numbers publicly released--$6-7 billion a year for "citizen biodefense"--do not include DoD, DHS or CIA figures, he declined to state what those figures might be.

In addition, as icing on top of the anthrax cupcake, the attacks were used to change existing biological weapons laws to grant the US government immunity from violating its own prohibitions, via The PATRIOT Act.

Add to the mix a top secret and nearly undetectable delivery system, plus the growing concerns about undesirable effects of a potential vaccine, and you've got a recipe for a biological weapons attack of massive proportions. Call it a pandemic and you're almost home free.

The one remaining step would be to launch a test to see how your world-changing mass murder event would play out in the real world. To do so without the incumbent casualties would seal the deal.

With its questionable lethality coupled with the global mechanisms now activated in response, it looks as if Covid-19 fits the profile.

We are now neck deep in the Big Muddy, so to speak. Whether other delivery systems will be activated soon, in order to transform Covid into "The Big One" or whether the way is being cleared for their later deployment, we are now submerged into a situation from which extrication is vital.

--March 17, 2020

36

LOCKDOWNS IN THIRD WORLD RESULT IN STARVATION, POLICE ASSAULTS

A number of developing countries which have initiated "Stay at Home" orders are now experiencing hunger and starvation deaths, as well as murders by over-zealous police.

Reports that the lockdowns in India and elsewhere have resulted in almost as many deaths as has the coronavirus are now emerging. A recent opinion piece in The Print discussed non-virus deaths in India which were a result of the loss of employment and loss of income, detailing these deaths as by starvation, suicide and assaults by security forces.[20]

The article states that "As India extends the lockdown in a modified form for another two weeks, here's another statistic we need to think about: at least 195 people have died of the lockdown." A number of examples are given of people dying due to the lockdown rather than the virus:

> "Enforced by the trigger-happy police officers through lathis, this lockdown has been so cruel it wouldn't even let ambulances pass in some places, such as in Mangalaru, where two people died as a result."

A reported assault by police on an ambulance driver resulted in another death.

> "In Maharashtra, the police assaulted an ambulance driver for allegedly ferrying passengers rather than patients. The officers took a bribe and let the ambulance go to the hospital so that the driver could be treated for assault injuries. The driver died anyway."[21]

India is not alone in experiencing starvation and security-related deaths. Ugandans are reported as also now facing the spectre of starvation as a result of attempts to curb the spread of the virus.[22]

A recent article in the Wall Street Journal also revealed that security forces in Uganda had killed people for defying the lockdown.[23] The Irish

Times also reported police beating civilians in Uganda, as part of their enforcement capacity vis a vis the virus.[24]

Police violence against civilians is also reported in Kenya, where the police recently beat to death a thirteen-year-old boy as part of their "crackdown" on the coronavirus.[25]

The situation in Latin America is not much brighter. The economies in many Latin American countries depend upon casual labor, and casual laborers generally don't have savings accounts. This makes compliance with social distancing and stay-at-home orders a recipe for starvation. As reported, a vegetable vendor in Haiti succinctly stated that "I am not going to spend money fighting corona. God is going to protect me."[26]

So far, the First World has been spared the spectre of starving neighbors and food riots. America has a considerable infrastructure to assist its needy, although there are now reports of food banks being stressed to their limits, as millions apply for unemployment benefits and other financial assistance.[27]

With the Third World going hungry and unable to respond vigorously to security-related attacks, one might want to revise the official perception that the elderly are the primary victims of Covid-19. It appears to be equally ravaging the poorer nations.

--April 14, 2020

37

COVID AND NURSING HOME DEATHS – THE CASE FOR INTENTIONAL GENOCIDE

A discussion of the genocidal potential for the Covid pandemic would not be complete without a hard look at its impact on the elderly. While Covid is reported to be far more dangerous for the aged, its impact on nursing home patients and the decisions leading up to the placement of Covid patients in these homes must be thoroughly dissected.

According to recent reports, somewhere between 30-50% of Covid deaths took place in nursing homes. New York Governor Andrew Cuomo's much discussed decision to place Covid patients into these facilities was preceded by statements from him acknowledging the peril posed by Covid spread in these homes. In an interview he conducted on March 10 with Jake Tapper, Cuomo stated "…that's my nightmare and that's where you're going to see the pain and the damage from this virus. Senior citizen homes, nursing homes, congregant senior facilities. That is my nightmare. We've taken steps, some drastic steps in this area, in New Rochelle, we're talking about. We said no visitors in a nursing home."

Cuomo went on to say, "All you need is 9-year-old Johnny to visit his grandmother in a nursing home, give her a kiss, and you can be off to the races. That's my fear. That population in those congregate facilities. That is really what we have to watch."[28]

However, on March 25, a scant two weeks later, Cuomo signed his infamous order directing nursing homes to accept "stable" Covid patients without testing them.

Let that sink in for a moment. Covid patients who were known to have had the virus but not tested to see if they still had the virus were put into homes known to be a petri dish for contagion.

As a result, Covid spread through these populations just as Cuomo had predicted, "like fire through dry grass." As of December 28, 2020, "A USA TODAY Network New York calculation of the confirmed and presumed deaths among New York nursing home residents according to the state COVID tracker found that the total ....was more than 7,600 ..."[29]

This statistic is misleading, however, as it does not include the numbers of nursing home patients who were transferred to and died in hospital. Those numbers are unpublished.

The State of New York rushed to exonerate Cuomo from culpability. A report issued by State Health Commissioner Dr. Howard Zucker insisted that the spread of the disease in nursing homes could be attributed to visitors, not to the stated policy of placing Covid patients in the homes. That policy was subsequently repealed.[30]

Other states have also reported significant numbers of nursing home deaths from Covid.

As reported in Healthline, "...Researchers reported that these facilities accounted for 63 percent of all COVID-19 fatalities in Massachusetts.

"They added that nursing homes also accounted for 81 percent of COVID-19 deaths in both Minnesota and Rhode Island at the time as well as 71 percent in Connecticut and 70 percent in New Hampshire.

"In another 22 states, long-term care facilities accounted for more than half of all COVID-19 fatalities."[31]

Another item of concern revolves around the fact that nursing home residents are dying due to lack of care rather than from the virus during this "public health emergency." As reported in the Associated Press, nursing home residents are now dying of dehydration and malnutrition, rather than from Covid, as homes are reportedly overwhelmed by the emergency. As the article states, "As more than 90,000 of the nation's long-term care residents have died in a pandemic that has pushed staffs to the limit, advocates for the elderly say a tandem wave of death separate from the virus has quietly claimed tens of thousands more, often because overburdened workers haven't been able to give them the care they need."[32]

The article goes on to report that "A nursing home expert who analyzed data from the country's 15,000 facilities for the Associated Press estimates that for every two COVID-19 victims in long-term care, there is another who died prematurely of other causes. Those "excess deaths" beyond the normal rate of fatalities in nursing homes could total more than 40,000 since March."

All of this would be simply tragic were it not for the fact that elderly people are already being targeted by government authorized guardianship programs as well as by euthanasia laws. The shocking legal abuses which have afflicted the elderly in these programs are now getting some mainstream coverage, though the articles generally posit that the problems are a result of a few "bad apple" guardians, rather than any concerted and systematic effort by the state to seize the assets and destroy the lives of those under guardianship.

One attorney, Ken Ditkowsky of Illinois, who was forcibly retired from the practice of law after over 50 years due to his attempts to protect the rights of a woman under guardianship, disputes this perception.[33] "This is a holocaust on the elderly," declares Ditkowsky. He has also been tracking the reports of nursing home Covid deaths, which he states further buttresses the argument that the elderly are on the chopping block.

A recent report from an advocate for guardianship reform, Teresa Kay-Aba Kennedy, reveals the intertwining nature of guardianship and Covid. In a report dated 1/09/2021, Kennedy writes,

"My 85-year-old mother is crying in the other room because she longs to hear her 92-year-old sister Lillie's voice. They are the last two siblings left of eight. Lillie is the matriarch of a family with upwards of fifty nieces and nephews. ALL of them have been blocked from even speaking with her for over four years after she was abducted by an improperly-appointed guardian and her own court-appointed attorney.

"Yesterday, we found out that the assisted living facility where Lillie has been in lockdown has multiple COVID-19 cases. When we called the local sheriff for a welfare check, the officer said he could not share any information stating that it violates HIPAA laws. We were told to contact the guardian who is not returning our calls and has unchecked power under current law. I called the State Ombudsman and his power seems to still be limited. No agency at the state or federal level seems to have the ability or the will to help. Last week, my mother filed yet another motion for visitation (with an emphasis on telephonic and video). Yesterday, the filing was returned indicating that the division had to be changed to Probate (versus Guardianship). Does this mean Aunt Lillie has died and no one told us?"

A number of states have scrambled to provide legal immunity to nursing homes. According to an article in the ABA, "At least 26 states, including Illinois, Michigan, New Jersey and New York, have implemented immunity provisions protecting long-term care facilities and other health care providers from civil negligence lawsuits arising from the COVID-19 pandemic – including decisions resulting from resource or staffing shortages."

Nevertheless, the article goes on to note that "There's no comprehensive database of case filings. But a COVID-19 complaint tracker posted on the website of the law firm Hunton Andrews Kurth shows 55 wrongful death lawsuits filed against long-term care facilities around the country as of early September. More suits are on the way, with plaintiffs attorneys in Florida, Massachusetts and other states that have mandatory presuit screening periods saying they are investigating and preparing to file cases."[34]

Euthanasia laws, or assisted suicide laws, also target the elderly and disabled. A number of states in the US have now passed these laws, including California, Colorado, District of Columbia, Hawaii, Maine, Oregon, Vermont and Washington. A New Jersey law is currently under appeal. A number of other states are currently considering the passage of assisted suicide legislation.

Add to the mix the existence of the "impostor" or "doppelganger" pharmaceuticals, packaged as your usual antibiotic or anti-anxiety medication or even potentially your Covid cure – these are black project pharmaceuticals which are known to cause cardiac arrest in the unsuspecting targets--and you have a recipe for even more deaths of vulnerable populations.[*]

–January 9, 2021

---

[*]   At the time of going to press, Biden's DOJ has announced it will not investigate the nursing home deaths attributed to Covid-19.

38

A DISTURBING ASPECT TO "SHELTER IN PLACE"

"Shelter in Place" may expose one to contamination.

Domestic legislation mandates a lack of transparency.

International treaties which should provide protection here are inadequate.

A number of years ago, an article appeared on Salem-news.com discussing the dangers of a "stay at home" policy should (and when) a pandemic occurs. The article specifically discussed the mounting concerns attached to revelations in blueprints that the government now has the capacity to selectively deliver a toxic substance into pre-selected homes, via the water lines.

The blueprints supporting this contention do not require an advanced degree in engineering to understand. There are now two main lines running down every street which are cross- connected via service lines. Whatever is in the second line can be pumped into pre-selected homes via the operation of a remote controlled valve, such as featured in the attachment.

This information has been heavily suppressed. Radio interviews, such as the one I did on the Alex Jones show a number of years ago, have been removed from websites. Contacts from disarmament groups, such as the Quaker American Friends Service Committee, initially voicing their alarm at what was presented in a series of articles concerning this critical infrastructure project, have suddenly been silenced. An editorial assistant at the *Los Angeles Times*, equally alerted to the significance of what I had uncovered, brought my work to the attention of the higher ups at the Times and was shortly thereafter let go.

It appears that work on this water project began in the US around the time that President "Tricky" Dick Nixon declared that the US was unilaterally abandoning its offensive biological weapons program. Shortly thereafter, the international treaty known as the Biological Weapons Convention came into effect, as other nations ostensibly concurred in the necessity to ban biological weapons. Research as yet unpublished indicates that Henry Kissinger, Secretary of State under Nixon, was heavily involved in reaching out to other countries in order to establish this water project elsewhere.

The unpublished research also has located the double line water system, aka water weapon, in Canada, Israel, Switzerland, post-invasion Iraq and in at least one capital city in Latin America. It is thought that this may be a woefully incomplete list.

This reporter has, under the mantle of an NGO, twice advised the Biological Weapons Convention in Geneva of these concerns. Responses by delegates to the Convention have confirmed the attention that has been paid to these presentations. However, the Convention is hamstrung by the legal anomaly of its failing to have executed a verification mechanism. Due to this, the Convention has no teeth and no ability to monitor or prosecute a violation of the Convention, which bans the development, production and stockpiling of biological weapons.

We are now entering a scenario where "Stay At Home" orders are not only being suggested and legally enforced, but also rewarded. "Snitches Get Rewards" claimed LA Mayor Gil Garcetti, as he advised people to turn in their neighbors for violating Covid-19 sequestration orders.

Whether or not the plan is to utilize the water weapon to further impact the viability of the pre-selected targets at this point in time—or at a later date– is not known.

Should a noxious chemical, rather than a biological agent, be pumped into your home via the water system in your city, the Chemical Weapons Convention would be the treaty that would have jurisdiction over the attack. However, the CWC has shown itself to be dedicated to accommodating the agenda of the United States on multiple fronts. The gas attacks in Douma, which CWC inspectors attempted to pin on Syrian President Assad, are being contested as US-generated machinations to unseat Assad.[22] Other, individual reports of chemical weapons attacks that could be traced back to the US are being summarily denied investigation by the CWC, which has stated that "The issue you mention in your e-mail falls under the remit of national authorities. Best regards."

In other words, "Gassed in Auschwitz? Complain to the Gestapo!"

The Critical Infrastructure Information Act of 2002 makes it a felony for US government employees to release information about critical infrastructure. This protection racket was furthered when President Trump signed CISA back in 2018, gutting any private right of action (a lawsuit) should anyone allege impropriety in the use or abuse of critical infrastructure.

Reports to DHS and the EPA about the dangers posed by a double line water system have been funneled into a "national-security" type of response. A recent public records act request to Winthrop, Massachusetts, concerning a water line project initiated in that city, was summarily and quite illegally ignored.

We appear to have been shut down in efforts to address these concerns through established channels. Given that the "Stay At Home" orders now in effect provide the desired platform for launching the water weapon (most people will be using their house water if they are confined to their homes), it is strongly advised to include water from outside the home on your prepper list. Store the water in your home and should you suspect that your tap water is contaminated, use the stored water.

A biological agent, such as Covid-19, which incurs a death rate of under 1%, is not the real danger here.[23] Crashing economies, mandated vaccines and your own house water may constitute a greater threat.

We are pretty much on our own here. It appears we have largely been abandoned by governments, media and ersatz human rights groups.

Water is life. It is your life and future at stake here. Be smart and take appropriate measures to protect yourself. Share this information with others and we will be able to get through this.

--April 17, 2020

39

THE SECOND VIRUS

"Who you are will overtake you. You become a monster so that the monster will not break you."

– U2, Peace on Earth

It is easy to delineate the name of the first virus, the one sweeping the globe, decimating whole economies and wreaking havoc on individuals, cultures and communities. This virus is said to have caused 2.3 million deaths worldwide and, if you believe the news, shows no signs of letting up.

Every day, we hear of new virus-connected horrors. It mutates and its mutations combine, thereby doing a clever detour around our best efforts to mitigate its impact, through our dedicated vaccination programs. The vaccines don't seem to work on the variants, which puts us back at the starting point. In fact, the vaccines may not protect us much at all. Pregnant women lose their babies, if not to the virus then to the vaccine. Our parents waste away, alone and abandoned, in the facilities into which we stuck them, never dreaming they would become hotbeds of infection. And when they expire in the homes, we may not even be told.

ANOTHER VIRUS

However, along with the coronavirus (corona means crown and is apparently aptly named) there is a second virus which has emerged. This virus has no name. Its genetic structure has not been isolated and its method of transmission is unclear. This virus attacks our souls.

It has attacked the conscience of our leaders, our news reporters and indeed anyone in a position of power. Once it has embedded itself at the apex of society, it proceeds in a downward spiral, infecting at random.

When Chris Hedges wrote the following, it highlighted the "trickle down" effects of this second virus on society at large and the involvement of those we have come to trust:

> We now live in a nation where doctors destroy health, lawyers destroy justice, universities destroy knowledge, governments destroy

freedom, the press destroys information, religion destroys morals, and our banks destroy the economy.

The second virus was first noted years ago in the conduct of those in the legal system, specifically lawyers and judges. Remember the "shark" jokes about lawyers? You can make the same jokes now about judges and prosecutors. It's become clear that the courts have gone off the rails and are involved in protecting certain kinds of behaviors, such as embezzlement and even murder, rather than routing out those committing these crimes and appropriately punishing them. This could not have been made more stunningly obvious than when Philip Esformes, convicted for using his position as nursing home owner to steal from not only his clients but from the government itself, was set free this past year only months following his imprisonment.

When it was disclosed that judges are regularly paid off, under the table, to throw cases this information was suppressed. The US Attorney's office in a number of states has been presented with facts supporting the conclusion that many judges are now regularly being covertly rewarded in a number of ways to execute the laws (pun intended) and every US Attorney's office that has been given this documentation has refused it.

The virus is also evident in the immunity granted police officers when they brutally attack or kill unarmed citizens. These same officers stood idly by as outraged Americans burnt down whole sections of cities in protest this past year. It has been suggested that they were ordered to do so.

This brings into focus how this virus functions. It functions by deferring responsibility for one's actions to others. "Acting under orders" is a favored mantra of those infected by the virus.

The attempt to attribute responsibility away from oneself and onto an authority is a chief attribute of the virus. It indicates that the virus is now fully embedded and has infected the individual who is in the process of denying his own humanity and his individual obligations as a human being.

This is how soul capture works. You're not responsible, or so you say.

There's Money To Be Made In Selling Your Soul

And while there is indeed money to be made in relinquishing your conscience, this is not the only mechanism at play. Being monetarily rewarded for abandoning your obligations to others is certainly a hefty temptation but not the only game in town. There is also the matter of one's personal protection and survivability.

It has been well documented that those held captive by criminals and terrorists tend to begin to identify with and serve their captors. The term, Stockholm Syndrome, refers to a 1973 high-profile hostage situation in which the hostages came to bond with their captors. After their release, the hostages refused to testify against their captors and began raising money for their defense.

According to *Heathline,*

> "With this syndrome, hostages or abuse victims may come to sympathize with their captives. This is the opposite of the fear, terror, and disdain that might be expected from the victims in these situations.
>
> Over the course of time, some victims do come to develop positive feelings toward their captors. They may even begin to feel as if they share common goals and causes. The victim may begin to develop negative feelings toward the police or authorities. They may resent anyone who may be trying to help them escape from the dangerous situation they're in."

Healthline goes on to report that "Many psychologists and medical professionals consider Stockholm syndrome a coping mechanism, or a way to help victims handle the trauma of a terrifying situation."

A TRAUMATIZED WORLD

If one accepts the conclusion that entire societies are now traumatized through the actions of their captors, otherwise known as "their leaders," one can begin to understand the psychological mechanisms that are turning whole societies into hostages and willingly obedient servants of problematic agendas. According to Nils Melzer, the UN Special Rapporteur on Torture, the preponderance of torture in so-called civilized societies can be traced to large -scale trauma. Melzer writes:

> The need to defend against threats to individual or public security is the predominant utilitarian basis upon which torture and ill-treatment are justified. One can see where the threats inherent first in the attacks of September 11 and now in the "public health emergency" of the pandemic would provide sufficient basis for the preconditions for torture cited here. (Report A/75/179 – E – A/75/179)

Inflicting torture and abuse is another sign of this second virus, the one that infects one's conscience and one's soul. There are now hundreds of thousands of individuals, world-wide, who claim to have been put into non-consensual weapons testing programs and are stating that they are being tortured through the use of these weapons against them. Some of these individuals have tracked their torturers to FBI Fusion centers and military operatives. Others are claiming that ordinary people, such as their neighbors, have been enlisted as torturers.

HITLER PAINTED ROSES

Those infected with the second virus may appear to be normal and may have "good" attributes. A sort of compartmentalization, common in trauma victims, may enable them to be "good citizens" and then turn into purveyors of lies, torture and abuse without an observable transformation.

It is commonly understood that humans are social animals and, as such, are open to social influence. Setting aside the financial rewards for betrayal and abuse for a moment, humans can be rewarded by social approval of their peers, or punished through shaming mechanisms. There is also potential for independent thought to be mitigated through chemical means, such as fluoridation, alcohol and psychiatric drugs.

However you frame it, betrayal and abuse are indicators of soul capture. For those resistant to the religious implications of that phrase, you can reframe it as "following orders," "going along to get along," or "the popular thing to do." It all equals the same thing. You've been infected by the second virus and are now a willing participant in the destruction of other people.

You can, however, recover.

It takes a dedicated effort to observe your own behaviors and to plumb the depths of your motives. It takes reconnecting with whatever you might want to call it – your higher self, your conscience, the Divine, the Universe. It takes deliberation and effort. It may not be easy. But for the sake of your own individual passage and for the sake of this endangered species called humanity, it may be the only route available. It may be uncomfortable and it may, in fact, be dangerous.

But consider the alternative.

--February 20. 2021

EPILOGUE

Epilogue

The articles in this book have revealed that the US has engaged in a gross manipulation of law, international accords, and human rights and has also taken a number of concrete actions which have brought us to today, where the entire world is now reeling from a biological agent. Several times in the narrative, I mentioned the situation in the Middle East and the possibility that another holocaust was pending and that a pandemic would figure in. That is, a selectively delivered pandemic.

The holocaust scenario is not a popular viewpoint at this juncture. Indeed, the growing incidents of violent anti-semitism plus a popularized contempt for Israel have indicated an upswell in anti-Jewish sentiment. Increasingly, Israel is seen as a powerful aggressor, victimizing the Palestinians in defiance of international law. While every President has claimed to be a friend of Israel, multiple authors are now disputing this as propaganda rather than reality. These include John Loftus, author of the 1994 bestseller, *The Secret War Against the Jews*, and others.

At the time of this writing, actions on the Middle Eastern stage support the previously stated concerns that the fate of Israel is married to the pandemic. It has been suggested that the ultimate release of a pandemic agent will be tied to a missile attack on the Jewish state.

In fact, technological advances may have trumped that initial perception. In May of 2020, it was reported in the Israeli and international news that Iran had attempted to hijack Israel's water systems and launch a poison attack through Israel's water. Through an assault on Israel coupled with a worldwide release of a pandemic agent through covert and selective delivery systems, a holocaust could be perpetrated and the actual culpable parties could appear non culpable. In closing therefore, we offer this recent article indicating that the capability for the destruction of Israel is right on schedule.

And as another indication of potential foul play, it must be remembered that Israel also has the water weapon capability, as revealed through Wikileaks secret cable releases.

40

Israel and Iran in Dead Heat Weapons Race

Israel is developing a laser weapons defense system that may end up neutralizing most of her airborne security threats.

The Iron Beam, which utilizes both ground based and air based platforms for a launch, was reported recently by the Israeli government to be in development and potentially ready to be tested later this year.[1]

And it may be not a moment too soon.

After President Trump backed out of the Iran nuclear deal, which had been signed by his predecessor President Obama, he chose to use sanctions as a method to force Iran into compliance. Iran responded by announcing that it was ramping up its nuclear development program. It is generally thought that Iran should have a working nuclear weapons capability within a year.[2]

Trump reportedly considered the Iran deal to be flawed and to facilitate Iran's nuclear development, which ended up taking place any way.

The Iron Beam, also reported to be possibly ready within the same time frame, would address the nuclear weapons threat. Iran has repeatedly threatened Israel with annihilation and recent aggressions between the US and Iran had commentators worried that we were heading for a direct confrontation.

In fact, rather than making Israel more secure, the US's repeated meddling in the region has resulted in far more vulnerability for the Jewish state.

Unlike President Obama, Trump has been touted as a friend to Israel. However, his acts of "friendship" have repeatedly resulted in more conflict between Israel and her neighbors. Trump's decision to move the US embassy from Tel Aviv to Jerusalem resulted in border clashes that left dozens dead. In a rather amazing act of revisionism, Trump recently denied that this violence took place. And his "Deal of the Century" peace plan has been roundly rejected by the Palestinians, who subsequently cut off diplomatic ties with the US and with Israel.

While the major media has continued to front the story that the US is a friend to Israel, the bald reality may be quite a bit different. While the US gives Israel over $3 billion a year in foreign aid, earmarked for purchasing weapons from the US, scrutiny of the reliability of some of these defensive weapons has resulted in concerns that the US is selling lemons to Israel.

According to research by MIT Professor Ted Postol, the much touted Iron Dome may not work.[3] David's Sling, also a defensive weapons system, has been reported as also problematic.[4] The final tier of Israel's defense system, the Patriot missile, is known to be junk.[5]

The US's complicity in Israel's growing endangerment is cautiously being discussed by a number of commentators. In an article in The Atlantic, former Ambassador to Israel Michael Oren writes that "Rather than a departure from long-standing policy, the hasty withdrawal of American troops from Syria appears to many in the Middle East as yet another American move that will strengthen Tehran."[6] Writing in the Jerusalem Post recently, Seth Frantzman was a bit more diplomatic when he stated that "An erratic Washington, even one that appears more pro-Israel than previous administrations, leaves more questions than answers. Israel's enemies exploit that kind of uncertainty."

It appears that within one year, Israel's race to construct an adequate defense system will bear fruit, or not. It appears that within the same time frame, Iran may finally be in a position to fulfill her promise to wipe Israel off the map. Either way, the US has been a silent partner in this unfolding saga.

--February 9, 2020

EXHIBITS

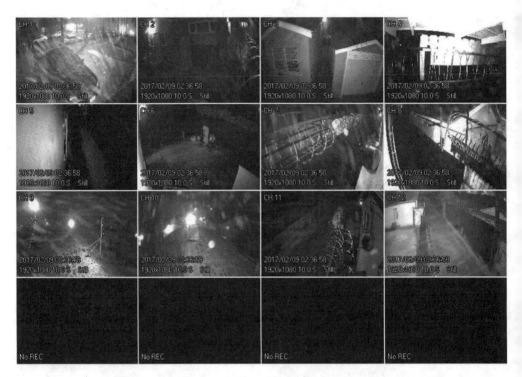

Exhibit A: Still from surveillance video on Los Angeles home.

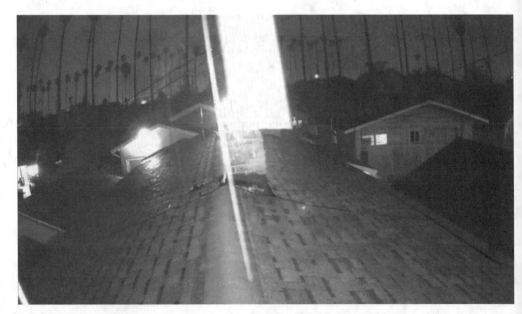

Exhibit B: Still showing laser/directed energy attack on Los Angeles home.

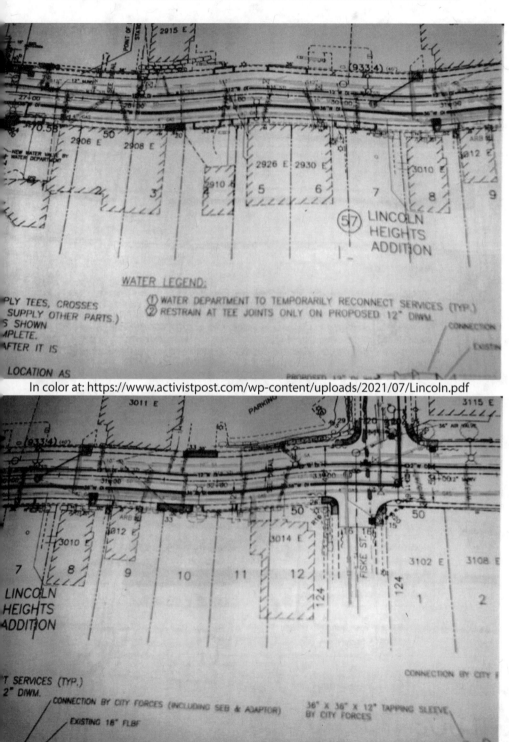

In color at: https://www.activistpost.com/wp-content/uploads/2021/07/Lincoln.pdf

Exhibits 1 & 2: Blueprints from Spokane water system.

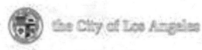

Department of Water and Power · the City of Los Angeles

ANTONIO R. VILLARAIGOSA
Mayor

Commission
H. DAVID NAHAI, President
EDITH RAMIREZ, Vice President
MARY D. NICHOLS
NICK PATSAOURAS
FORESCEE HOGAN-ROWLES
BARBARA E. MOSCHOS, Secretary

RONALD F. DEATON, General Manager

November 21, 2006

Ms. Janet Phelan
Mt. Baldy Lane #1
Sandpoint, Idaho 03894

Dear Ms. Phelan:

Subject: California Public Records Act (CPRA) Request: Los Angeles Department of
Water and Power (LADWP) Ardmore Avenue Area Cement Lining Project.

This letter is a follow-up to our letter to you dated October 30, 2006, regarding your CPRA
request dated and received October 23, 2006, which sought records relating to the
Los Angeles Department of Water and Power's Ardmore Avenue Area Cement Lining
Project.

Additional records are now available for your review.

Please be advised, however, that some of the documents available have been partially
redacted because some information contained in the requested records is exempt from
public disclosure due to the security-sensitive nature of the information. California
Government Code Section 6255 provides public agencies the right to withhold any records
if the public interest of non-disclosure clearly outweighs disclosing the information.

You also requested information regarding "remote-controlled" valves used in the project.
There were no such valves used in the project.

To schedule a viewing of the records now available for your review, please contact the
LADWP CPRA Coordinator at (213) 367-4440. During the record review session, you may
indicate which, if any, records you wish to have photocopied. In accordance with the
Los Angeles Administrative Code, the fee for this records duplication service is $1.00 for
the request, 10 cents per 8.5x11-inch or 8.5x14-inch page, and 25 cents per 11x17-inch
page. There is no fee if you wish only to review the documents. Payment, which is due at
the time of the request, may be in cash or check made payable to Los Angeles
Department of Water and Power.

Water and Power Conservation ...a way of life

111 North Hope Street, Los Angeles, California 90012-2607   Mailing address: Box 51111, Los Angeles 90051-5700
Telephone: (213) 367-4211 Cable address: DEWAPOLA

Exhibit 3: Two-page letter from Los Angeles Department of Water and Power

Ms. Janet Phelan
Page 2
November 21, 2006

You will be notified approximately every two weeks as additional records become available.

If you have any additional requests for records, you are encouraged to submit your request on the LADWP CPRA Request Form, a copy of which is enclosed. A written request helps clarify the records being sought and will assist us in our response to you. LADWP CPRA Request Forms are available at the LADWP website www.ladwp.com/ladwp/cms/ladwp006433.pdf or from the CPRA hotline at (213) 367-4440.

Sincerely,

Ronald F. Deaton
General Manager

Enclosure

Office of the City Attorney
City Hall
1685 Main Street
PO Box 2200
Santa Monica, California 90407-2200

City of
Santa Monica

August 8, 2006

Ms. Janet Phelan
81 Mount Baldy Lane, #1
Sandpoint, Idaho 83864

Re: Public Records Request

Dear Ms. Phelan:

This letter is in response to your public Records Act request direct to the City Attorney's Office and the Public Works Department Dated July 27, 2006.

After careful review, the City finds that the two (2) requests seek information and documents that are highly sensitive and jeopardize the security of the City.

Your request to the Public Works Departments seeks:

1. Copies of all contracts with private companies and or person doing work on the Water Main Replacement Project, etc.

    Response: The Public Works Department responds by stating that the documents requested are highly sensitive in nature and are not discloseable under Section 6255. You inaccurately identify Section 6254.8 as the information being discloseable. The construction and application is for salaries of individually identifiable public employees.

2. Copy of this agency's written guidelines for accessibility of records under the California Public Records Act, etc.

    Response: The City invokes the California Public Records Act as its guideline.

tel: 310 458-8331• fax: 310 395-6727

Exhibit 4: Two-page letter from City of Santa Monica.

August 8, 2006
Page 2

Your Request to the Office of the City Attorney seeks:

1. Copies of all Documents, if any, which demonstrates that blueprints for the Water Main Replacement Project, etc.

   Response: The City responds by stating that the documents requested are highly sensitive in nature and are not discloseable under the California Public Records Act (CPRA) Section 6254 (a), (f) and (k). To delineate the exceptions, the City identifies materials which are expressly exempt from disclosure, (a) interagency or intra-agency memoranda which are confidential to protect the security of the City; (f) security files, (k) federal law-Homeland Security Act of 2002.

   The City also invokes Section 6255 as the catchall exception which permits the government agency to withhold records if it can demonstrate that, on the facts of the particular case, the public interest is served by withholding records clearly outweighing the public interest served by disclosure. Government Code §§6254 et seq. and §6255, Gilbert v. City of San Jose (App. 6 Dist. 2003) 7 Cal. Rptr. 3d 692. The Act recognizes that certain records should not, for reasons of privacy, safety and efficient governmental operation, be made public. Haynie v. Superior Court, 26 Cal.4th 1061 (2001).

The City has a legitimate concern for safety and efficient governmental operation. To reiterate it to you, compelling the City to produce blueprints to water mains exposes the public to extreme dangers to the security of the water supply. Producing this information would cause severe risks to the safety and welfare of the public. Therefore, it is necessary and critical that we deny your request.

We would like to assist you and we will provide reasonable access to any documents which are readily identifiable and available for disclosure, if any exist. Gov. Code §6253.1 and §6254 (k).

Sincerely,

JOSEPH LAWRENCE
Assistant City Attorney

By:

Eugenia Jiménez
Community Liaison

cc: Gil Borboa, EPWM
    Carlos Rosales, EPWM
    Robert Martinez, SMPD

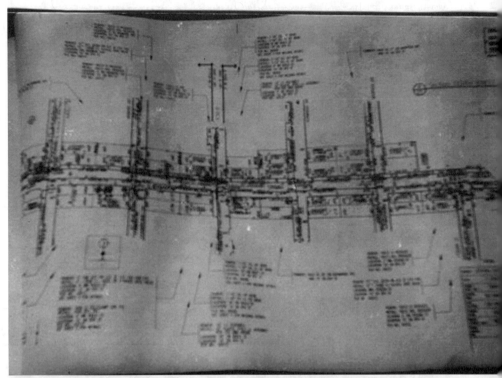

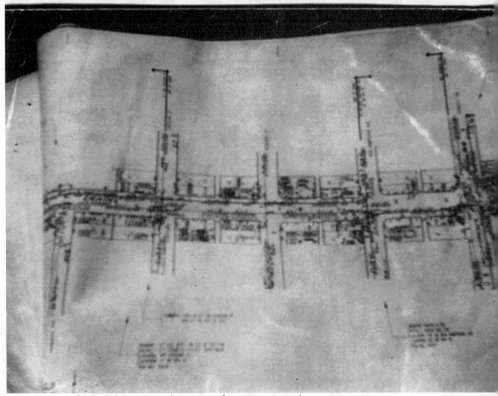

Exhibits 5&6: Blueprints from Los Angeles water system.

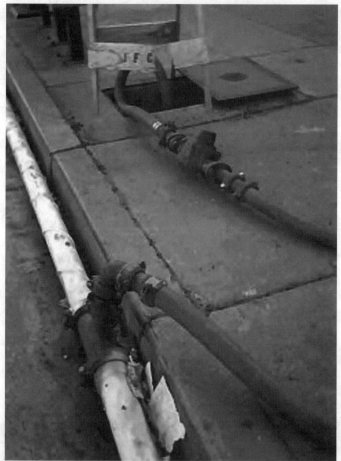

Exhibit 7: Gutter line bypassing water lines during construction work.

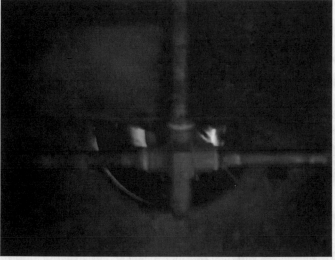

Exhibit 8: A tee joint, enabling the flow of water North/South and East/West

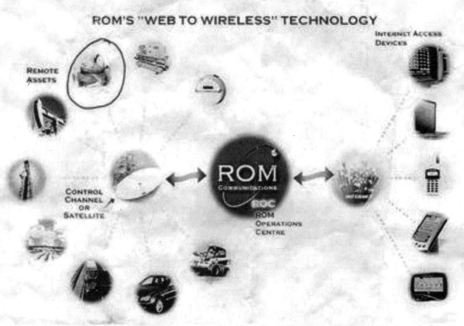

Exhibit 9: ROM Communications diagram, showing how a water valve (top left) can be impacted by signal from a cell phone or laptop

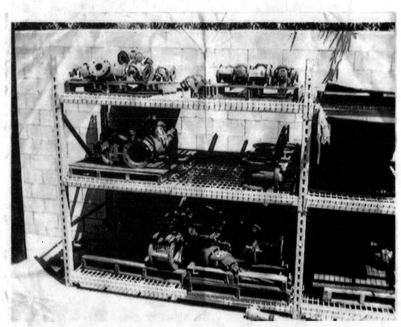

Exhibit 10: Gate valves with RFID addresses stacked up in Santa Monica City Yard.

City of
Santa Monica®

Office of the City Attorney
City Hall
1685 Main Street
PO Box 2200
Santa Monica, California 90407-2200

April 28, 2004

Janet Phelan
1616 7ᵗʰ Street
Santa Monica, California 90401

Re: <u>Public Records regarding Work on Water Lines</u>

Dear Ms. Phelan:

The City has evaluated your request and responds by informing you that there are no documents responsive to your request.

The Public Records Act is to be administered liberally by the City to facilitate the disclosure of records. However, facilitating research is not the purpose of public access to government records under the California Public Records Act. (Gov.Code Sections 6254, 6254 (k) and Section 6255). Moreover, the Act recognizes that certain records should not, for reasons of privacy, safety and efficient governmental operation, be made public. <u>Haynie v. Superior Court</u>, 26 Cal.4th 1061 (2001)

Sincerely,

JOSEPH LAWRENCE
Assistant City Attorney

By: _[signature]_
EUGENIA JIMENEZ
Community Liaison

cc: Gil Borboa, EPWM Utilities

tel: 310 458-8336 • fax: 310 395-6727

Exhibit 11: Letter from City of Santa Monica stating there are no water line work records.

ENDNOTES

SOME BACKGROUND

1.   https://www.washingtonpost.com/wp-dyn/content/article/2011/02/15/AR2011021502251.html

2.   https://www.usatoday.com/story/news/nation/2014/09/22/biolab-safety-incidents-lassa-fever-h7n9-burkholderia/15908753/

3.   https://www.usatoday.com/story/news/nation/2014/09/22/biolab-safety-incidents-lassa-fever-h7n9-burkholderia/15908753/

4. https://www.activistpost.com/2012/01/dancing-apocalypso-with-microbial.html

5. https://www.gq.com/story/colin-powell-walter-isaacson-war-iraq-george-bush

6. http://www.osan.af.mil/news/story.asp?id=123449327

7. http://koreajoongangdaily.joins.com/news/article/Article.aspx?aid=3013044

8. https://www.theguardian.com/world/2015/jul/14/come-and-see-our-pesticide-factory-its-not-for-anthrax-says-north-korea%20%20%C2%A0

9. http://www.defense.gov/Portals/1/features/2015/0615_lab-stats/docs/USD-Frank-Kendall-Action-Memo-to-DSD-on-the-Results-of-the-Comprehensive-Review.pdf

10.   https://www.usnews.com/news/articles/2012/12/24/global-flu-pandemic-inevitable-expert-warns

11 http://neworleans.indymedia.org/news/2007/05/10214.php

12. https://www.brookings.edu/blog/up-front/2020/06/16/race-gaps-in-covid-19-deaths-are-even-bigger-than-they-appear/

13. https://www.activistpost.com/2012/01/dancing-apocalypso-with-microbial.html

14.   https://www.nytimes.com/2012/10/12/world/panetta-warns-of-dire-threat-of-cyberattack.html

15.https://www.monsanto.com/products/pages/roundup-safety-background-materials.aspx

16. https://www.huffingtonpost.com/tamar-haspel/condemning-monsanto-with-_b_3162694.Html

17.   http://www.naturallysavvy.com/eat/whats-so-bad-about-gmos-top-ten-reasons-to-avoid-them#sthash.OU6DEqKJ.dpuf

18.http://www.journal-neo.org/2015/08/23/us-water-systems-may-be-used-for-a-wmd-attack/

19. http://www.gewater.com/

20 https://www.sec.gov/rules/other/35-27539.htm#P250_39637

21 http://www.rwe.com/web/cms/en/113648/rwe/press-news/press-release/?pmid=766

22 https://www.dailymail.co.uk/news/article-1200004/Did-MI5-kill-Dr-David-Kelly-Another-crazy-conspiracy-theory-amid-claims-wrote-tell-book-vanished-death.html

STATE OF THE SCIENCE

1. https://www.technocracy.news/cambridge-scientists-create-artificial-embryos-from-stem-cells/

2. https://www.theguardian.com/science/2003/apr/14/genetics.research

3. http://www.usa-anti-communist.com/ard-blog/Ethnic_Biological_Weapons.php

4. https://www.youtube.com/watch?v=r0PdVa5gxoA

5. https://www.activistpost.com/2018/07/thousands-of-scientists-sign-pledge-against-developing-lethal-a-i.html

6. https://www.activistpost.com/2018/07/darpa-mind-control-troops-weapons.html

7. http://www.activistpost.net/bwcreport%20ithaca.pdf

8. https://www.activistpost.com/2017/08/lies-damnable-lies-downright-dangerous-lies.html

9. https://crispr.synthego.com/?gclid=CLmrzd_R5s0CFUokhgod7IkHRw%20

10. https://techcrunch.com/2016/07/08/jennifer-doudna-inventor-of-gene-editing-technology-crispr-cas9-is-coming-to-disrupt/

11. https://www.dni.gov/files/documents%20/SASC_Unclassified_2016_ATA_SFR_FINAL.pdf

12. http://www.hfea.gov.uk/index.html

13 http://www8.nationalacademies.org/onpinew/newsitem.aspx?RecordID=12032015a

14. https://aeon.co/essays/can-parents-be-trusted-with-gene-editing-technology

15. http://www.sculptingevolution.org/genedrives

16. https://en.wikipedia.org/wiki/Exclusionary_rule

17. https://www.govtrack.us/congress/bills/110/s1858

18. http://www.projectcensored.org/top-stories/articles/16-human-genome-project-opens-the-door-to-ethnically-specific-bioweapons/

19. http://www.idf.org/regions/africa/about

20. http://www.voanews.com/content/diabetes-sub-saharan-africa-africa-hopeclinic-projecthope/1554338.html

21. https://vimeo.com/6484188

22. https://www.theguardian.com/politics/2013/jul/16/david-kelly-death-10-years-on

23. http://www8.nationalacademies.org/onpinews/newsitem.aspx?RecordID=12032015a%C2%A0

24 https://www.nature.com/nature/journal/v528/n7580_supp/full/528S7a.html

25. https://www.theguardian.com/science/2015/dec/01/human-gene-editing-international-summit%20%20%C2%A0

26. https://www.theguardian.com/science/2015/dec/04/human-gene-editing-is-a-social-and-political-matter-not-just-a-scientific-one

27. https://www.businessinsider.com/china-edited-human-genome-laws-2015-4%C2%A0

28. https://www.nih.gov/about-nih/who-we-are/nih-director/statements/statement-nih-funding-research-using-gene-editing-technologies-human-embryos%20

29. http://www.npr.org/sections/health-shots/2014/04/10/301432633/scientists-publish-recipe-for-making-bird-flu-more-contagious

30. http://journals.plos.org/plospathogens/article?id=10.1371/journal.ppat.1006390

31. http://www.npr.org/sections/health-shots/2017/06/15/532925945/just-small-genetic-tweaks-to-chinese-bird-flu-virus-could-fuel-a-human-pandemic

32. https://www.reuters.com/article/us-health-birdflu-mutations-idUSKBN1962ID

33. http://www.cidrap.umn.edu/news-perspective/2015/07/cdc-dod-anthrax-errors-involved-575-shipments

34. https://www.babysfirsttest.org/newborn-screening/newborn-screening-legislation

35. https://edition.cnn.com/2010/HEALTH/02/04/baby.dna.government/index.html

36. https://www.fbi.gov/services/laboratory/biometric-analysis/codis/ndis-statistics

37. https://www.schneier.com/blog/archives/2012/10/protecting_and.html

38. https://www.armyupress.army.mil/Journals/Military-Review/Directors-Select-Articles/Ethnic-Weapons/fbclid/IwAR2UJ1YoqssWu-o1tJ7kwioLTom_Pcko-YkYEXFWfEC-Zv950av6H9w5G0TQ/

39. https://journal-neo.org/2014/06/03/doctor-who-ran-biowarfare-unit-faces-sentencing/

40. https://www.modernghana.com/news/900528/why-the-us-government-hits-africa-with-ebola.html

41. https://fas.org/irp/threat/cbw/nextgen.pdf

42. https://kcnawatch.org

43. http://www.firedoglake.com/2015/01/25/a-lost-document-from-the-cold-war-the-international-scientific-commission-report-on-bacterial-warfare-during-the-korean-war/

44. http:/cryptome.org/2015/01/isc-biowar-kr-cn.pdf

45. http://english.hani.co.kr/arti/english_edition/e_international/694269.html

46. http:/www.cbrneportal.com/interview-with-dr-peter-emanuel-the-joint-united-states-forces-korea-portal-and-integrated-threat-recognition/%20 %C2%A0

47. https://abcnews.go.com/Politics/pentagon-inadvertently-shipped-live-anthrax-labs-states/story?id=31346018%C2%A0

CREEPING TOWARDS FASCISM

1. http:/fas.org/news/iraq/1998/12/21/981221-scott.htm

2. https://www.newyorker.com/magazine/2004/05/10/torture-at-abu-ghraib

3. https://en.wikipedia.org/wiki/Doctors%27_trial%20

4. https://www.nytimes.com/1994/04/11/us/cold-war-radiation-test-on-humans-to-undergo-a-congressional-review.html?pagewanted=all

5. https:/www.whitehouse.gov/the-press-office/2010/11/24/presidential-memorandum-review-human-subjects-protection

6. http://medicalkidnap.com/2015/05/16/medical-kidnapping-in-the-u-s-kidnapping-children-for-drug-trials/#sthash.igT60zk3.dpuf

7. http://www.pharmpress.com/files/docs/paeditaric_sample_chapter.pdf

8. http://www.medicalkidnap.com/2016/01/12/arizona-mom-loses-battle-to-regain-daughters-medically-kidnapped-pleads-for-someone-to-adopt-them/

9. https://www.businessinsider.com/electronic-warfare-weapons-2012-3%20

10. http://www.projectcensored.org/wp-content/uploads/2010/05/ElectromegnaticWeapons.pdf

11. http://www.edgewoodtestvets.org/press-releases/pdfs/20160202-MoFo-Wins-Another-Ninth-Circuit-Victory-For-Veterans.pdf

12. http://www.fas.org/sgp/clinton/humexp.html%C3%A7

13. http://america.aljazeera.com/opinions/2015/12/has-obama-banned-torture-yes-and-no.html

14. http://www.edgewoodtestvets.org/

15. http://www.sosbeevfbi.com/mystory.html

16. https://www.theatlantic.com/business/archive/2015/02/for-great-american-cities-the-rich-dont-always-get-richer/385513/%C2%A0

17. http://www.chicagotribune.com/news/ct-chicago-lead-water-risk-met-20160207-story.html

18. http:/www.nytimes.com/2016/02/09/us/regulatory-gaps-leave-unsafe-lead-levels-in-water-nationwide.html?_r=0

19. http://www.thefreethoughtproject.com/navajo-water-supply-horrific-flint-cares-native-american/

20. http://articles.philly.com/2016-02-06/news/70376889_1_lead-exposure-lead-problem-blood-lead-level

21. http:/www.ibtimes.com/political-capital/hillary-clinton-spotlighting-crisis-flint-michigan-voted-against-measure-prevent

22. https://www.nytimes.com/2013/04/11/health/parents-of-preemies-werent-told-of-risks-in-study.html?_r=0

23. http://www.psychcrime.org/news/index.php?vd=986&t=Psychiatrist+Derek+A.+Ott%2C+reprimanded+in+patient+death%2C+received+%2494K+from+pharma+companies+

24. https://www.activistpost.com/2010/12/10-modern-methods-of-mind-control.html

25. http://www.republicbroadcasting.org/news/chloramine-causing-collateral-health-damage/

26. http:/www.webmd.com/a-to-z-guides/features/drugs-in-our-drinking-water

27. http://events.jspargo.com/sso16/Public/Enter.aspx

28. http://www.wcrf.org/int/cancer-facts-figures/data-cancer-frequency-country

29. https://en.wikipedia.org/wiki/Death_and_state_funeral_of_Jack_Layton

30. https://www.activistpost.com/2013/11/youve-met-edward-snowdennow-meet.html%20

31. http://www.foxnews.com/printer_friendly_wires/2008Nov19/0,4675,MarylandPoliceSurveillance,00.html

32. http://www.defense.gov/Portals/1/features/2015/0615_lab-stats/Review-Committee-Report-Final.pdf

33. http://www.sltrib.com/home/2563809-155/utah-lab-that-shipped-anthrax-has

34. https://www.congress.gov/bill/114th-congress/senate-bill/2383/text%C2%A0

35. https://www.activistpost.com/2017/08/lies-damnable-lies-downright-dangerous-lies.html

36. http://www.activistpost.net/170731SupplementalPoliceReport.pdf

37. http://www.projectcensored.org/car-powered-water-idea-mysteriously-dies-inventor/

38. https://www.theatlantic.com/politics/archive/2013/03/killing-americans-on-us-soil-eric-holders-evasive-manipulative-letter/273749/

BIOWEAPONS: AT THE BREAKING POINT OF HISTORY

1. http://www.huffingtonpost.com/2014/05/01/smallpox-related-virus-georgia-orthopoxvirus-_n_5247288.html

2. https://www.activistpost.com/2011/06/concerns-continue-to-mount-on-us.html#%21bkLSjM

3. https://www.muckrock.com/foi/united-states-of-america-10/cold-death-chemical-weapons-and-means-of-mass-destruction-11476/

4. https://www.activistpost.com/2012/01/dancing-apocalypso-with-microbial.html

5. https://www.theguardian.com/world/2014/oct/03/-sp-ebola-outbreak-risk-global-pandemic-next

6. http://blogs.shu.edu/ghg/2012/01/06/ruminations-on-the-seventh-review-conference-of-the-bwc-more-or-more-of-the-same/

7. http://www.state.gov/secretary/rm/2011/12/178409.htm

8. http://www.unog.ch/80256EDD006B8954/%28httpAssets%29/570C9E76CAAB510A-C1257972005A6725/$file/ADVACNCE-BWC+7RC+Final_Document.pdf

9. http://www.thewednesdayreport.com/articles/research/weapons_of_mass_destruction-super_diseases.htm

10. http://www.unog.ch/80256EDD006B8954/%28httpAssets%29/4192F51D1A8D7C2E-C1257965004A4EFC/$file/ITHACA.pdf

11. http://articles.sfgate.com/2008-05-05/news/17153864_1_critical-care-task-force-health-care

12. http://www.cbw-events.org.uk/rg.html

13. https://journal-neo.org/2015/06/29/just-say-anything-the-us-responds-to-the-un-review-of-its-human-rights-record/

14. https://www.activistpost.com/2012/01/dancing-apocalypso-with-microbial.html

15. https://documents-dds-ny.un.org/doc/UNDOC/GEN/N04/561/49/PDF/N0456149.pdf?OpenElement

16. https://undocs.org/S/AC.44/2013/17

17. https://sputniknews.com/world/201609081045088663-us-russia-biological-laboratories/

18. https://www.strategic-culture.org/news/2016/09/03/russia-questions-peaceful-nature-us-biological-research.html

19. https://www.armscontrol.org/factsheets/cwcglance

20. https://portswigger.net/daily-swig/dhs-to-overhaul-cybersecurity-ops-through-creation-of-cisa

THE PANDEMIC

1. https://www.theguardian.com/commentisfree/2020/apr/06/coronavirus-free-speech-hungary-fake-news

2. https://www.greenmedinfo.com/blog/dr-fauci-nejm-editorial-suggests-covid-19-fatality-rates-may-be-10x-lower-official

3. https://www.rollingstone.com/politics/politics-news/doj-suspend-constitutional-rights-coronavirus-970935/

4. https://www.smdp.com/california-cities-want-transparency-rules-waived-in-pandemic/188672

5. https://www.cnbc.com/2018/06/28/wealth-transfer-baby-boomers-estate-heir-inheritance.Html

6. https://www.youtube.com/watch?v=EyDQdeYYx_I

7. https://www.americanprogress.org/c3-our-supporters/

8. https://www.forbes.com/sites/brucelee/2020/09/26/what-is-the-death-rate-for-covid-19-coronavirus-what-this-study-found/?sh=7731363f5c46

9. https://www.techtimes.com/articles/252203/20200901/fauci-slams-cdc-new-low-statistics-showing-6-covid-19.htm

10. https://www.express.co.uk/news/uk/1331999/UK-lockdown-coronavirus-test-leeds-middlesborough-tynside-corby

11. https://economictimes.indiatimes.com/industry/healthcare/biotech/healthcare/controversial-vaccine-studies-why-is-bill-melinda-gates-foundation-under-fire-from-critics-in-india/articleshow/41280050.cms

12. https://www.activistpost.com/2015/08/us-water-systems-may-be-used-for-a-wmd-attack.html

13. https://www.activistpost.com/2013/07/questions-arise-as-to-coroners-cover-up.html

14. http://www.spiraxsarco.com/learn/modules/6_1_01.asp

15. https://www.popularmechanics.com/military/a49/1227842/

16. http://articles.latimes.com/2012/jul/08/nation/la-na-biowatch-20120708

17. http://www.dhs.gov/xlibrary/assets/nipp-ssp-water-2010.pdf

18. https://www.theguardian.com/world/2014/oct/03/-sp-ebola-outbreak-risk-global-pandemic-next

19. https://nationalinterest.org/blog/buzz/coronavirus-vs-flu-which-worse-130782

20. https://theprint.in/opinion/more-than-300-indians-have-died-of-the-coronavirus-and-near-ly-200-of-the-lockdown/400714/

21. https://www.hindustantimes.com/cities/covid-19-probe-ordered-into-ambulance-driver-s-death-after-assault-by-policeman/story-45pj0d8MHMh4uudCnribWP.html

22. https://www.nytimes.com/reuters/2020/04/01/world/africa/01reuters-health-coronavirus-uganda.html

23. https://www.wsj.com/articles/in-africa-fierce-enforcement-of-coronavirus-lockdowns-is-stirring-resentment-11585825403

24. https://www.irishtimes.com/news/world/africa/no-beating-on-patrol-with-the-ugandan-

military-enforcing-curfew-1.4227963

25. https://www.irishtimes.com/news/world/africa/coronavirus-anger-over-excessive-violence-by-kenyan-police-1.4218135

26. https://abcnews.go.com/International/wireStory/coronavirus-hits-rich-poor-unequally-latin-america-69874281

27. https://www.zerohedge.com/health/breadlines-erupt-across-america-lockdowns-crush-americas-working-poor

28. https://www.governor.ny.gov/news/audio-rush-transcript-governor-cuomo-guest-cnns-lead-jake-tapper-0

29. https://www.dailyadvent.com/news/604f1d56e79cd6065bb9ed101d98d148-Nursing-home-death-toll-remains-elusive-but-it-is-certainly-higher-than-official-total

30. https://nypost.com/2020/07/06/cuomos-nursing-home-edict-not-to-blame-for-deaths-report/

31. https://www.healthline.com/health-news/covid-19-racing-through-nursing-homes-what-families-can-do

32. https://apnews.com/article/nursing-homes-neglect-death-surge-3b74a-2202140c5a6b5cf05cdf0ea4f32

33. https://journal-neo.org/2014/03/28/us-moves-to-crush-internal-dissent/

34. https://www.abajournal.com/magazine/article/coronavirus-related-deaths-in-nursing-homes-seed-lawsuits-and-questions-about-whos-responsible

35. https://ahtribune.com/world/north-africa-south-west-asia/syria-crisis/3180-opcw,-douma-and-the-post-truth-world.html

36. https://nypost.com/2020/03/31/covid-19-death-rate-lower-than-previously-reported-study/

37. https://www.healthline.com/health/mental-health/stockholm-syndrome#definition

EPILOGUE

1. https://www.timesofisrael.com/defense-ministry-announces-breakthrough-in-anti-missile-laser-development/

2. https://www.wired.com/story/how-close-is-iran-to-a-nuclear-weapon-heres-what-we-know/

3. https://www.technologyreview.com/s/528991/an-explanation-of-the-evidence-of-weaknesses-in-the-iron-dome-defense-system/

4. https://www.jpost.com/Arab-Israeli-Conflict/Wheres-Davids-Sling-and-why-wasnt-it-used-to-intercept-Irans-missiles-578377

5. https://foreignpolicy.com/2018/03/28/patriot-missiles-are-made-in-america-and-fail-everywhere/

6. https://www.theatlantic.com/ideas/archive/2019/11/israel-preparing-open-war/601285/

The following articles originally appeared in *Activist Post*:

Pandemic Watch: Another Insider Announces that a Global Pandemic is Imminent, January 2013

Things that go bump in the night: Keeping Skippy safe from the Terr'ists, October 2012

Bayer Buys Monsanto — More To This Merger Than Meets The Eye, September 2016

Porton Down's Legacy of Death: Inquest to Take Place Shortly Concerning Death of Scientist, May 2013

Lawsuit Seeks Injunction Against EPA "Gas Chamber" Experiments, May 2012

The Strange Convergence of Technologies of Life and of Extermination, July 2018

Genetic Weapons–Can Your DNA Kill You?, June 2013

How To Kill a Whole Lot of People: Scripps Scientists Publish How They Made H7N9 Virus More Transmissible, June 2017

The US Wants Your DNA: The Dark Underside of Genetics, October 2019

Cancer, Cancer Everywhere … But Not In The Presidential Suite, October 2019

Chemical Weapons Allegedly Used Against Political Target in Los Angeles, August 2017

Dancing the Apocalypso with the Microbial Gestapo, January 2012

US Lies to UN Concerning Weapons Status (Originally titled Lies, Damnable Lies and Downright Dangerous Lies) August 2017

Trump Signs Bill to Further Protect Critical Infrastructure, Including Pandemic Delivery System, November 2018

Justice in the Time of Corona, April 2020

Is Covid-19 "The Big One" Or Just A "Dry Run?," March 2020

Lockdowns in Third World Result in Starvation, Police Assaults, April 2020

Israel and Iran in Dead Heat Weapons Race, February 2020

The following articles originally appeared in *New Eastern Outlook*:

The Biological Weapons Convention Turns 40, May 2015

The Anthrax Files: US Forces Conducted Multiple Secret Anthrax Experiments in South Korea, December 2015

MIT States That Half of All Children May be Autistic by 2025 due to Monsanto, January 2015

Doctor Who Ran Biowarfare Unit Faces Sentencing, June 2013

Gene Editing: The Dual-use Conundrum, July 2016

First GMO Corn, then Frankenfish, and Now — Get Ready for Designer Babies, December 2015

North Korea Blasts U.S. for Germ Warfare Program, July 2015

Human Experimentation Rampant in the United States, March 2016

US: Torture Without Borders, September 2016

Going Beyond the Obvious Horror: Lessons From Flint, Michigan, March 2016

Former FBI Anthrax Investigator Files Lawsuit Claiming Retaliation, June 2015

DoD's Final Report on Anthrax Fiasco a Whitewash. January 2016

Book Review: The 2001 Anthrax Deception (Originally titled US Biodefense: A Wolf in Sheep's Clothing) September, 2014

Smallpox: A Deadly Shell Game, July 2014

Bioweapons: At the Breaking Point of History, August 2016

US Water Systems May be Used for WMD Attack, August 2015

Articles originally published in *The Americans Bulletin*:

Water as a Weapon, (July/August 2007)

Articles Originally published in *Salem-News*:

Homeward Bound, February 2011

Articles Originally published in *Communal News*:

A Disturbing Aspect to Shelter in Place